What Are You Doing to Your Body?

*Thirteen Simple Changes Can Make
the Rest of Your Life
the Best of Your Life*

Alon Biran NC

iUniverse, Inc.
New York Bloomington

iUniverse books may be ordered through booksellers or by contacting:

iUniverse
1663 Liberty Drive
Bloomington, IN 47403
www.iuniverse.com
1-800-Authors (1-800-288-4677)

Because of the dynamic nature of the Internet, any Web addresses or links
contained in this book may have changed since publication and may no longer be
valid. The views expressed in this work are solely those of the author and do not
necessarily reflect the views of the publisher, and the publisher hereby disclaims
any responsibility for them.

ISBN: 978-1-4401-7829-0 (sc)
ISBN: 978-1-4401-7827-6 (hc)
ISBN: 978-1-4401-7828-3 (ebook)

Library of Congress Control Number: 2009911918

Printed in the United States of America

iUniverse rev. date: 01/11/10

Contents

Acknowledgements

I'd like thank first and foremost my best friend, wife and the mother of our two baby boys for putting up with me during the long and sometimes arduous process of writing this book.

I'd also like to thank all those who have been instrumental in helping to bring this book to fruition.

My dear friend Samuel Noris for coming through with the beautiful artwork.

Susan Capparelli from Write For You, who is responsible for the initial editing of the first draft of this book and for steering me in the right direction.

To my friends and family who offered advice when I needed it.

To Tal Hermalin for your help with the graphics.

And finally to everyone at iuniverse for making sure this book adheres to the highest standards.

Thank you all

Introduction

Who Are You, Alon Biran,
and Why Should I Read Your Book?

Ever since I can remember, I was always attracted to nature. From a flower that mimics the appearance of a bee in order to attract bees to the exact timing of birds' migration, I was fascinated by the perfection of nature; nothing in nature is accidental.

Later in life this attraction led me to look to nature when faced with disease or discomfort. I always believed that Mother Nature is the best pharmacy on earth and that nature has the best remedy to any imbalance either through proper nutrition or by the use of healing herbs. And so I began reading hundreds of books and attending numerous lectures on the subjects of natural healing and nutrition. Later on I attended the Global College of Natural Medicine and graduated with honors.

One thing that became quite apparent to me as I was delving into the world of health and nutrition is that most books offered a certain philosophy and a lifestyle that was based on this particular philosophy—and usually one philosophy contradicted the other.

Some examples of these philosophies are the zone diet, the raw food diet, and macrobiotics, as well as some ancient philosophies like traditional Chinese medicine and Ayurveda, the five-thousand-year-old Indian system of medicine. However, I found that although some principles deeply resonated with me, it was very difficult to adapt the entire philosophy to modern-day living. For example, try to eat nothing but raw food when you work as a salesperson constantly on the run or cook Indian food for hours every day if you'd like to apply the principles of Ayurveda.

Over time I found that instead of trying to adapt to one philosophy, I can collect the principles that resonate with me and seem to apply to the modern-day lifestyle from each philosophy. These principles served me well even when living a hectic New York City life and can be applied practically by anyone, no matter where you are in life and how healthy you are.

I believe that although the book you are about to read doesn't offer a new philosophy, it does offer a set of principles never before collected into one book, that can apply to anyone, anywhere and set any individual on the road to a healthier living.

The core guideline that leads these principles is *nature*; we always have to remind ourselves that humans are first and foremost mammals. According to National Academy of Science, all mammals, including humans, share 92 percent of their DNA.[1]

---

[1]   www.koshland-science-museum.org

Most principles that apply to other mammals should also apply to humans. As a result I always ask myself, would I be able to adopt a certain principle if I was a cave man? How did our ancestors behave? What did they eat? How did they heal?

We may like to think that we are very different than our ancestors, but the reality is that although we have evolved somewhat in the last fifty thousand years, biologically and physiologically we are not very different than the first *Homo sapiens*. However, our lifestyle has transformed dramatically, especially in the last 150 years or so. And so the challenge is to take those principles that worked for humans for thousands of years and apply them to modern-day living. And that is exactly what this book and the thirteen principles it presents aim at doing.

These principles have helped me to stay healthy when everyone around me comes down with the flu. By applying these principles I was able to avoid a dangerous operation on my back to remove a herniated disk and treated it naturally. They have also helped my clients to resolve many medical imbalances, from being overweight to other chronic conditions. But as my mentor T. Harv Ecker likes to say, *"Don't believe a word I say."* I would urge you to try these principles for yourself and see that they also work for you.

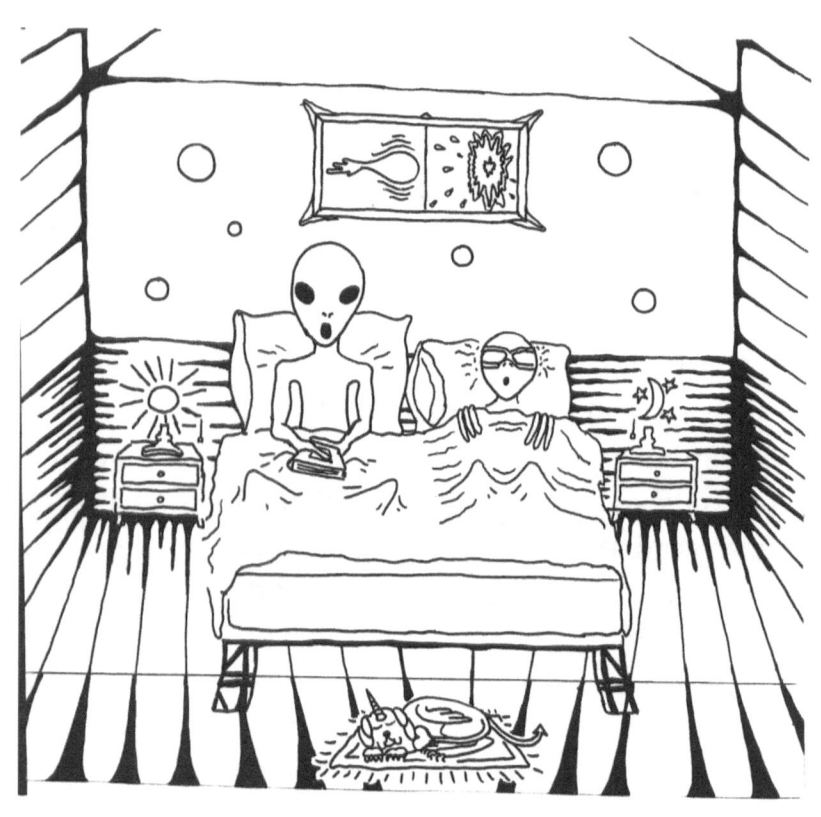

Wife: *What happened?*

Husband: *I bought this book and it's for humans only! Do you think I can get my money back?*

First Thing First

It is health that is real wealth and not pieces of gold and silver.
—Mahatma Gandhi

All human beings living on earth have five things in common (and if you are not one, you should pick up another book!). We arrive on this planet by birth, leave it by death, and in between we eat, drink, and breathe in order to survive.

Life on earth is a journey, a trip we all take. Our body is the vehicle for this trip, and our soul is the driver. When we are first born our body is like a brand new $300,000 Ferrari. As we age our Ferrari gets older and needs more maintenance and regular tune-ups. Every once in a while we have to see a mechanic, in the form of a medical doctor.

If you bought a $300,000 Ferrari that required the highest quality fuel as well as constant maintenance and tune ups in order to perform at its peak, would you neglect this precious baby of yours? Would you feed it only regular fuel, change its oil once every thirty thousand miles at best, and give it no other fluids?

How well do you think it would perform after a year? Two years? Five?

Your body is a much more sophisticated, delicate, and precious vehicle than any luxury car. And unlike your vehicle, which you can replace every three to five years, your body is with you for life. The only time you get to replace it is when you pass on. Why travel for most of life's journey in a broken-down vehicle?

This book highlights thirteen simple changes you can make to ensure the rest of your life is a healthier one. It's never too late to begin.

As the ancient Chinese text, the Tao Te Ching says, "Even the biggest problem in the world could have easily been solved when it was still small."

What that means in relation to your health is that preventing disease from manifesting in your body in the first place is the best and easiest way to enjoy a healthy life. And the earlier we start, the better off we are.

However, living in a healthy manner does *not* mean just having a Caesar salad every once in a while. Rather, it's an entire lifestyle you commit to consciously. The food you eat, the liquids you drink, and the air you breathe all play a role in how well your body performs. And while we all slip up occasionally, it's important to get back on track quickly.

One more tip before you begin reading. Each chapter contains practical information and tips you can implement in your daily life. However, as with any new habit, it takes time to implement new ideas and get used to them. Therefore, I highly recommend reading only one chapter a week, or even one a month. This will allow you the time you need to assimilate and put into practice the suggested ideas and exercises.

Finally, before you delve into the pages of this book, I'd like to offer a quick disclaimer. The information presented here is based on my own knowledge and experiences and includes concepts that work for me. I in no way claim that these are the best, or only, ways of doing things. As you read through the book, use your own judgment to decide if the recommendations are right for you. And experiment with the principles described to see what works in your own life.

Here, then, are thirteen practical and effective principles that can really help you to reach old age with a body (or vehicle) that is full of energy, agility, and verve.

Chapter 1

Eat What Nature Intended

Nothing will benefit human health and increase the chances for survival of life on Earth as much as the evolution to a vegetarian diet.
—Albert Einstein

Let's take a step back from the daily rat race for a moment and look a little more closely at ourselves. Do you realize that we are really just upright apes with extremely developed brains? That's right, according to The American Museum of Natural History, genetically our DNA is a 98.8 percent match with chimpanzees![2] And what do these close cousins eat? Let's have a look:

1. Orangutan: Living in the treetops of the rainforest of Indonesia, this large, gentle red

---

2   The American Museum of Natural History in New York City, 2009 Hall of Human Origins/ www.amnh.org/exhibitions/permanent/humanorigins/past/dna.php

ape is one of our closest relatives, sharing 97 percent of the same DNA as humans. Their diet is made up of bark, leaves, flowers, a variety of insects, and most importantly, over three hundred kinds of fruit.[3]

2. Gorilla: Gorillas are predominantly herbivores, eating mostly plant material. They forage for food in the forests during the day. They eat leaves, fruit, seeds, tree bark, plant bulbs, tender plant shoots, and flowers. They have been known to eat various parts of over two hundred different plant species. Occasionally, gorillas supplement their diet with termites and ants.[4]

3. Chimpanzee: Chimpanzees are omnivores (eating plants and meat). They forage for food in the forests during the day, eating leaves, fruit, seeds, tree bark, plant bulbs, tender plant shoots, and flowers. They also eat termites, ants, and small animals (they have even been known to eat young monkeys).[5]

A close look at these diets tells us that our closest relatives thrive predominantly on plants, roots, and fruits, supplementing occasionally with animal source protein in the form of prey or insects. It only makes

[3]   www.orangutan.com
[4]   www.enchantedlearning.com
[5]   www.enchantedlearning.com

sense that what is good for our closest relatives should be good for us.

Eat Fresh

Fresh fruits and vegetables are rich in living enzymes that are vital for proper digestion of food. In addition, they contain vitamins, minerals, and anti-oxidants essential to our health and longevity, as well as fiber that is crucial for intestine health. I can't stress enough the importance of eating at least one large serving of fresh fruits and/or vegetables every day.

Mother Nature has designed a perfect kitchen for us, one that offers the right food at the right season. However, in the United States and other Western countries some fruits and vegetables are available year-round thanks to globalization.

Nevertheless, choosing fruits and vegetables in season and locally grown can be extremely beneficial. With every day that elapses from the time a fruit or a vegetable is picked at the field or orchard, to the time it reaches your plate it loses its freshness and vitality. This means you receive fewer enzymes, vitamins, and minerals.

And where can you buy locally grown fruits and vegetables? At farmers' markets; most large cities now operate farmers' markets, and they are a great source for locally grown produce. If you can't get to a farmers' market, one way of knowing when fruits and vegetables are in season is watching their price; when the price drops you know the produce is in season. For example, the price of berries drops by almost half between end of April to end of June, and you should cash on it.

Other staples of the modern diet are grains and legumes (beans). These impose a challenge on modern-day diets for dietitians and nutritionists alike, as most of them endorse these foods as being super-foods and extremely beneficial to our health.

The reality, though, is that if you were dropped in a middle of a wheat or rice field without means of igniting fire, you would not be able to consume these foods. However, if you were extremely hungry, you would have been able to chew their sprouts. According to Dr. Joshua Rosenthal, head of The Integrative Institute of Nutrition in New York City, most legumes and grains are seeds and as such contain phytic acid in the outer layer of the barn, which makes them hard to digest. This is nature's way to protect these seeds from being eaten by animals before they had a chance to sprout.

However, once they sprout this phytic acid breaks down, and it becomes easier to digest these grains or legumes. The conclusion is that grains and legumes have to be consumed after they are sprouted, a process that occurs after they have been soaked in water for a few hours. If you were to examine the way traditional people eat legumes, you would realize that they always soak them in water for at least twelve hours, and even restaurants who serve legumes usually soak them for a few hours, which is good news. When it comes to grains, it is much harder to find sprouted products, although they do exist—mostly in health food stores.

My recommendation is that whenever you cook legumes such as beans, lentils, chickpeas, and green peas at home, you should soak them first for at least eight hours. You can do the same with many grains such as rice, oats, quinoa, barley, etc. As far as bread, it's best to avoid it unless you can find sprouted bread, which is available in health food stores and even in some supermarkets.

The Meat of It All

This brings me to one of the most controversial areas of nutrition today. The debate of whether we were supposed to eat meat or not has raged in the nutrition world for decades. My view in this respect is that biologically and structurally we were not designed to consume meat. Our jaw can move from side to side in order to grind but carnivores' jaws can only move up and down for tearing and biting. A carnivore's teeth are sharp and pointed for killing and tearing up prey, but we have molars for crushing and grinding. A carnivore's intestines are three times the length of its trunk, allowing meat to move through quickly so it won't rot. Ours are twelve times the length of the trunk, designed to extract as much nutrients as possible from fibrous food such as fruits, roots, and vegetables. I'll get back to this point a little later.

However, over thousands of years we have probably adjusted to consume animal-based protein in moderate quantities. The fact that our closest natural relatives, chimpanzees, do so, as well as the fact that we rely on animal products for vitamin B12 and the argument that early humans shed their hair and developed more sweat glands in order to out-run animals (see chapter 4, "Running") all point in this direction.

Here's the problem with meat, though; as seen in the movie *Fast Food Nation,* the animals (that includes beef, pork, and fowl) whose meat we are consuming are in large part grown in commercial farms in inhuman, crowded, sedentary conditions (and that is a social conscious issue as well). They are injected with hormones to speed up their growth and antibiotics to prevent infections. And you ingest all of this when you eat their meat—the hormones, the antibiotics, the fat of an animal that didn't move much and was living in its own manure and worst of all, the emotions of fear and anxiety of an animal that was living in grave conditions before it went to be slaughtered.

That brings me back to the length of our intestines; our intestines are designed to digest large amounts of fiber but are not designed for meat consumption and extraction. When you eat a diet that is rich in animal protein and lacks fiber, some portions of meat tend to get stack to the intestinal walls, rot, and ferment. This rotten meat fragments lead to growth of bacteria and infection inside the intestines, which later can lead to colorectal cancer, the second deadliest form of cancer.

As a matter of fact, a large federal study of AARP members published recently at Archives of Internal Medicine found that people between the ages of fifty and seventy one years old who consumed on average 4.5 ounces of red meat per day increased their chances of dying from heart failure 31 percent for men and 50 percent for women. For processed meat, the highest intakes of 1.5 ounces per day were associated with a 16 percent overall increased risk of dying in men and 25 percent increased risk in women. Cancer risk was about 20 percent higher in those who ate the most red meat, and 10 percent higher in those who ate the most processed meats.[6]

The Organic Way to Eat

After reading this chapter I hope that you'll reach the same conclusion as I have: the proper diet for those of us seeking health, longevity, and vitality should consist of fruits, vegetables, root vegetables, and nuts in abundance, grains and legumes in moderation, and unless vegetarian, meat (preferably organic and/or grass fed) or fish once or twice per week. Wild-caught fish is the best option, as it's free of saturated fat and

---

[6] Meat Intake and Mortality: A Prospective Study of Over Half a Million People, Sinha et al. *Arch Intern Med.*2009; 169: 562–571

is loaded with essential fatty acids (more on fats in chapter 7).

I also highly recommend choosing organic whenever possible. Organic food is free of herbicides, pesticides, hormones, and antibiotics and contains more vitamins and minerals than non-organic food. When you choose organic food you not only help your own body but you also make a statement on a much larger scale about maintaining earth's biodiversity, which is so essential for the rest of our existence.

> You can obtain a shopper's guide to pesticides in produce that lists the *Dirty Dozen* and the *Clean 12*— the best and worst produce in relation to pesticides. It is highly recommended that you consume the produce listed as *Dirty Dozen* organic. To obtain the list go to www.foodnews.org.

For those of you who shy away from organic food because of its price, keep this in mind; the more you and other people buy organic food, the less it will cost. In addition, most big supermarket chains now offer organic options at a cost very similar to non-organic food. So, the next time you buy non-organic food, think of all the deadly, toxic chemicals you're ingesting. Then consider that for just a few pennies more per pound you can have food that is completely clean and more potent.

Want more incentives? I promise you'll see the payback in reduced medical bills over the years to come.

Getting in the Habit

The next time you visit the supermarket, pay attention to what's in your cart. Is it mostly fresh, raw fruits and vegetables or frozen and processed food?

If it is mostly frozen and processed food, turn back to the vegetable aisle. Try to tip the balance in favor of fresh produce (and that doesn't include salads made up of iceberg lettuce in plastic bags).

If your cart already contains a good portion of fresh produce, pay a visit to the organic food area. Compare the prices with the non-organic food. Once again, try to tip the balance in favor of a larger portion of organic produce.

If you eat fresh food, brimming with energy and vitality, you'll quickly feel your own energy and vitality surge as well.

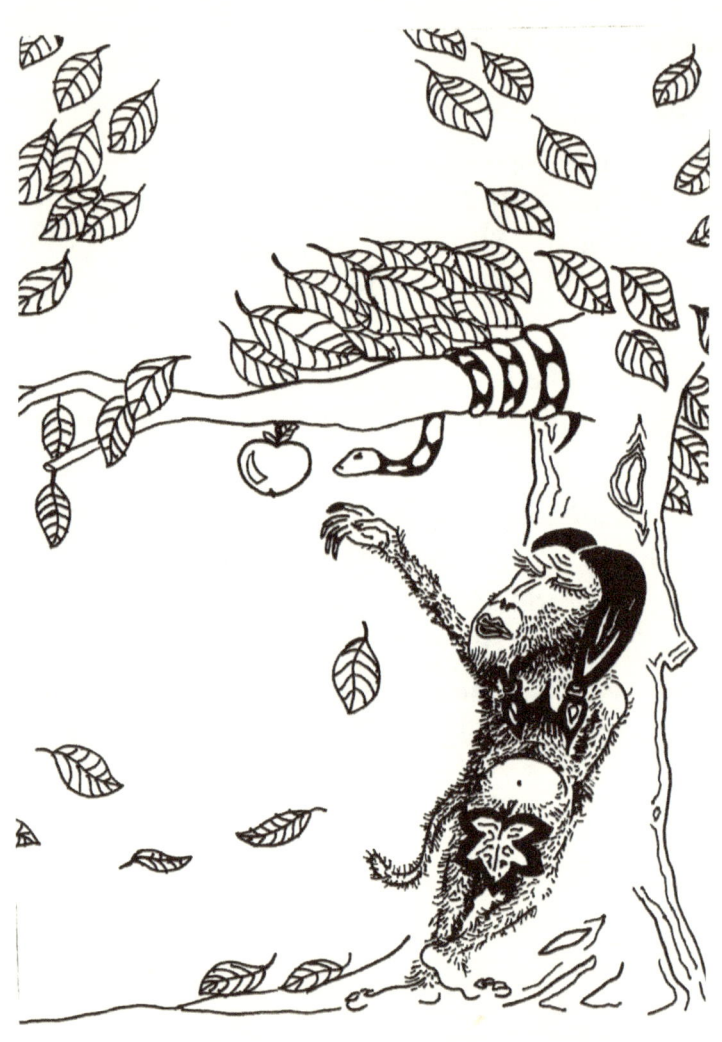

Sorry Ms. Ape, no salami today,
you'll have to eat the apple

Chapter 2

Refrain from Refined

I don't eat junk foods and I don't think junk thoughts.
—Peace Pilgrim (Mildred Lisette Norman)

Unfortunately, most of the food around us in supermarkets is "white poison" (i.e., pre-packed, refined, or processed foods). It's the process of refining and processing foods like flour, rice, and sugar that depletes them of their vitamins, minerals, and the dietary fiber that is so instrumental in keeping our colon clean.

All carbohydrates we digest turn into sugar in the form of glucose before entering the bloodstream. When we eat wholesome, unprocessed food packed with vitamins, minerals, and dietary fiber, it takes our digestive system time to break down all these nutrients. When we eat refined and processed food, however, it not only lacks most the nutrients of unprocessed food but also converts into glucose more rapidly. This is because the digestive system doesn't have to do the extra work to break down all these additional nutrients.

The result is a fast but unsustainable rise in blood sugar levels, prompting the body to secrete massive amounts of insulin, the hormone responsible for delivering glucose to the various cells. Massive insulin secretion leads to sudden crash in blood sugar levels, which, in turn, leaves us famished and fatigued. Now we're craving even more sugar, which only exacerbates the conditions of unstable sugar levels in our blood.

The Roller-Coaster Effect

The effect of this roller-coaster ride is that we are constantly craving more food, especially sweets and noncomplex carbohydrates. The latter are carbohydrates like white bread, pizza, and pastries that have been stripped of their nutrients.

If we continue this vicious, chaotic cycle we begin to gain weight. This is because the only cells that will continually accept glucose, regardless of how much energy was spent, are the storage bins of our body—the fat cells. But even worse than that, we may cause our cells to become resistant to insulin, resulting in the infamous syndrome X insulin resistance—a precursor to type 2 diabetes. And diabetes is one condition we all want to stay away from.

The Low-calorie Swindle

Even using low-calorie products like Equal, Splenda, and different diet sodas contributes to this vicious cycle. Artificial sweeteners not only affect your blood sugar levels, increasing your appetite and causing you to crave more sweet foods but also contaminate and poison your blood, cells, and ultimately the liver. According to Dr. Sandra Cabot MD, author of several bestselling books, including the *Liver Cleansing Diet, The Body Shaping Diet, Don't Let Your Hormones Ruin Your Life,* and many more, when you ingest aspartame, the main ingredient in most artificial sweeteners, it is absorbed from the intestines and passes directly to the liver via the liver filter. The liver breaks down or metabolizes aspartame to its toxic components—phenylalanine, aspartic acid, and methanol. The process of metabolizing aspartame to its toxic components requires a lot of energy from the liver, which means there will be less energy remaining in the liver cells. The result of this ordeal is that the liver cells will have less energy for fat burning and metabolism, which will ultimately result in fat storing.

According to the Global College of Natural Medicine, the artificial sweetener aspartame, which is the technical name for some well-known brand names, such as NutraSweet, Equal, Spoonful, and Equal-Measure, is one of the most dangerous substances added to food on the market today.

Aspartame is responsible for over 75 percent of adverse reactions to food additives reported to the U.S. Food and Drug Administration (FDA). Many of these reactions are very serious, including seizures and death. There are thirty-five symptoms and illnesses related to aspartame, among them headaches/migraines, seizures, weight gain (yes, weight gain!), depression, insomnia, anxiety attacks, memory loss, brain tumors, multiple sclerosis, Parkinson's disease, diabetes, Alzheimer's, and birth defects, just to name a few. And the alternative artificial sweetener, saccharin, used in Sweet'n Low, has been on the government's list of known or suspected carcinogens since 1977.

The solution is to use wholesome, complex carbohydrates such as brown rice, legumes, and whole-wheat products. These wholesome products contain the necessary vitamins, minerals, and other nutrients in the outer shell, which wasn't removed through processing, thus it takes the body longer time to metabolize them and they release to the blood stream in a slower manner. As a result, consuming these wholesome products will make you feel more satisfied after a meal, keep your blood sugar balanced, and reduce your cravings.

The "All Natural" Fraud

Beware, though, of products that pose as "all natural" or wholesome. The best example is whole wheat or multi-grain breads. Although containing whole wheat or multi-grain, many of these products also contain an abundance of additives such as food colorings, sugar (in the form of corn syrup or evaporated cane juice), and preservatives. To best of my knowledge, bread should only contain wheat (preferably whole wheat), grains, yeast, water, and a pinch of salt. Any other ingredient is meant to enhance the taste and shelf-life at the expense of your health.

As to the biggest modern-day consumer fraud, the combination words *"all natural,"* folks, almost any ingredient in food is "natural." Chemicals are natural, gasoline is natural, and poisons are natural too. If I may be a bit blunt and graphic, our own manure is natural too. It doesn't mean that we eat it though! Don't fall for this marketing scheme. The only way to ensure a product doesn't contain harmful ingredient is by reading the label, and certified organic food is usually safe too.

Satisfying Your Sweet Tooth

When you've just got to have it a little sweeter, whether it's food or a drink, use unrefined stevia (a natural sweetener available at health food stores), honey, agave nectar, or real maple syrup. These natural sweeteners enter and break down in the blood more slowly, resulting in a more sustainable rise in blood sugar levels.

The golden rule—always check the labels of products you intend to buy. If you can't pronounce the names of the ingredients on the package or if they contain aspartame, put it back on the shelf.

Getting in the Habit

For the next week carefully check the ingredients in every product you intend to buy. If their labels contain additives, preservatives, food coloring, and other long, strange, unpronounceable names, put that item back on the shelf and search for a simpler alternative. Also, beware of the ingredients *corn syrup* and *evaporated cane juice* (organic or not). These are just more appealing names for refined sugar.

Also, pay attention to the number of sweetened drinks you consume throughout the day. Every week try and cut it down by one serving a day. If you consume three sweetened drinks per day, next week cut back to two and the following week to one. After a month or so your consumption should be down to *zero* ... and that's a mighty healthy choice.

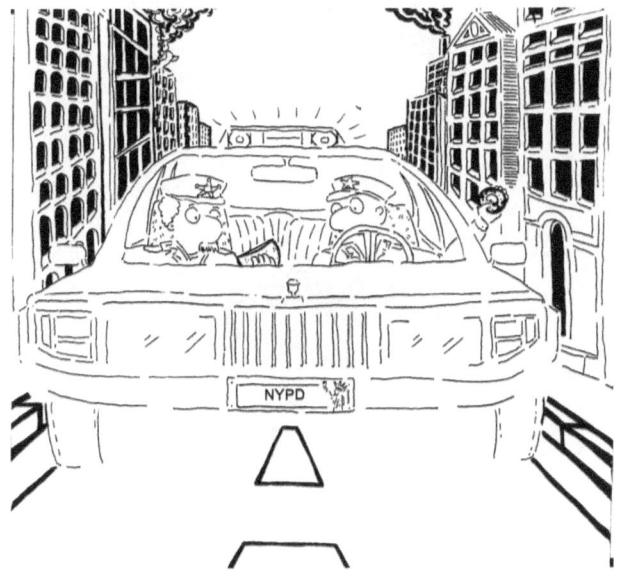

Cop A. *What are you eating?*

Cop B. *Whole wheat pita bread.*

Cop A. *Why?*

Cop B. *I'm reading this book that says donuts are not good for you.*

Cop A. *So why pita bread?*

Cop B. *It's still round, ain't it?*

Chapter 3

The Art of Food Combining

Healthy people care how they feel after a meal
as much as they care how the meal tastes.
—*Brian Tracy, Self-Help Expert*

Each mammal species on earth has a unique digestive system, one biologically adapted to a particular type of food. The lion's digestive system is different from the zebra's, and the cow's is different from the bear's. There are carnivores, herbivores, omnivores, and other vores living on earth.

Scientists can't seem to agree what type of digestive system human beings possess. One thing is certain, though, even though *we can't possess them all,* we insist on eating the diet of the lion, the cow, the ape, and defiantly, the pig. And usually all in one meal.

According to Daniel P. Reid, author of *The Tao of Health, Sex & Longevity,* just as some people don't get along, so some types of food don't mix well. The different types of food we eat are assimilated by different digestive juices and enzymes in different parts of the digestive tract. For example, carbohydrates require alkaline digestive juices such as the enzyme ptyalin and their breakdown begins in the mouth, while fruits assimilate in the intestines. Proteins, on the other hand, break down in the stomach and require secretion of pepsin and a highly acidic medium, in a process that takes about four hours.

When we combine these different food groups into one meal, the different digestive juices with contradicting PH levels neutralize one another. The result is a weak, watery solution in the stomach that digests none of the food groups and leaves us fatigued, unnourished, and bloated. It also clogs our intestines, making us sick.

When you add water or soft drinks to meals, it further neutralizes the digestive system, impairing digestion.

The Correct Food Combinations

Fruits

Fruits are very easy to digest and as such are impatient and rush to the intestines. This means they should not be mixed with any other food and are best eaten on an empty stomach. It makes them a great choice for breakfast or appetizers and a lousy choice for dessert. When you eat fruit, either right before or right after other foods, they get stuck in your stomach instead of reaching the intestines immediately as they should. The result is their fermentation, which, in turn, leads to excess gas, bloating, and yeast infestation.

Carbohydrates and Startch

Carbohydrates such as legumes (beans & peas), grains; including bread, pasta, and rice, potatoes, sugars, and pastries require mostly alkaline digestive juices and cannot be combined with animal-based proteins that require mostly acidic digestive juices. However, they make a great combination with vegetables and/or fats.

Some may wonder why I am cataloging legumes (beans, lentils, and peas) as carbohydrates, which are not supposed to be mixed with animal-based proteins as they themselves contain protein. Indeed, legumes are rich in both carbohydrates and protein. However, the proteins legumes contain differ in their structure, density, and digestibility from animal-based protein; the latter is much more dense and harder to digest. This makes legumes a great source of plant based protein.

The same goes for nuts, which can be categorized as fats but are also rich in protein and as a matter of fact are the best source of protein for the human body with pecans and almonds leading the pack, to the attention of all you bodybuilders out there.

Proteins

Animal-based proteins such as meat, poultry, fish cheese, and eggs (require acidic digestive environment) shouldn't be eaten with carbohydrates (starch or sugars) or fats at the same meal. Sorry, no steak and potatoes or eggs and home fries. It is also advisable to avoid mixing two kinds of proteins in the same meal. So, no bacon and eggs or ham and cheese.

Fats & Vegetables

Well, there is hope. Fats, such as vegetable oils, butter and nuts, can be combined with either carbohydrates or vegetables (more on fats in chapter 7). And vegetables go with everything; they're rich in enzymes that aid digestion. So it is very important to eat a lot of raw vegetables every day. You see, it's not all bad.

The tomato paradigm; many people consider tomatoes to be vegetables and use them a lot in salads. However tomatoes are closer to fruits in their consistency and PH composition.

Therefore it is recommended consuming tomatoes on their own and not combining them with carbohydrates or proteins. Since I don't know too many people who enjoy biting into a beef-steak tomato as if it was an apple, and most people do take joy of adding tomatoes into their salads, my recommendation is to eat tomatoes sparingly and mostly during the summer months. When consuming tomatoes try and do so as part of a vegetable salad without adding carbohydrates or proteins.

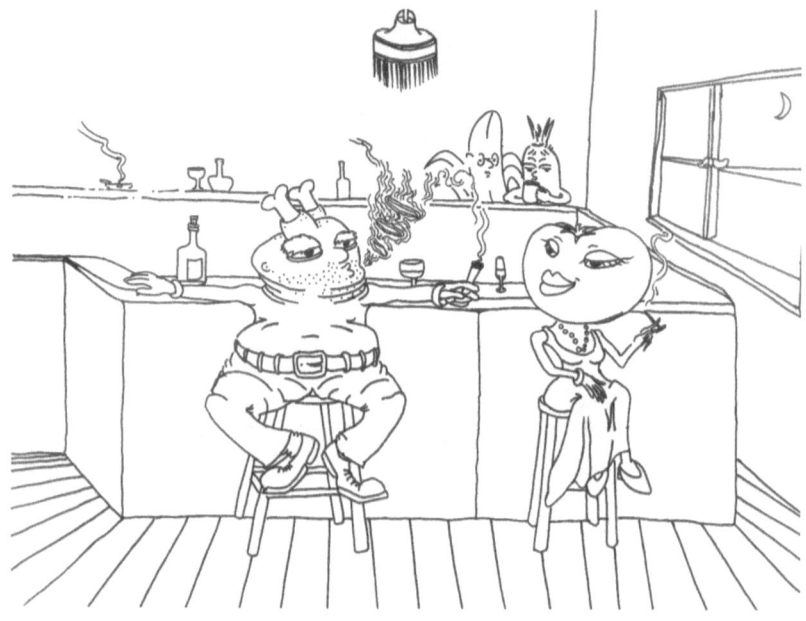

Carrot: *I can't believe tomato is going with him*
Cucumber: *Ah, don't worry, she's a fruit*
Carrot: *So...*
Cucumber: *So, fruits are kindda snobbish, she'll never go with the meat!*

The Liquid Dilemma

Now we come to the important topic of liquids. Just as you shouldn't drink and drive, you should also refrain from drinking and eating at the same time. I know many people find this instruction hard to follow, as they feel they need to wash down the food they eat with liquids.

Here's what happens when you gulp liquids while you eat. Water has a neutral PH. This means that it neutralizes the gastric juices needed to digest the food you eat. If it is soda or fruit juice you drink, that just adds sugar to the mix. Either way, the result is fermentation, bloating, and undigested food going through your system. This can cause autointoxication and yeast infestation in about 90 percent of the American population.

Candida albicans is a parasitic, yeast-like fungus that thrives in warm-blooded animals. Normally, it co-exists harmoniously with other micro-flora in the warm, inner creases of the digestive and vaginal tracts. *Candidiasis* or *yeast syndrome* is a complex medical syndrome that occurs when the balance between the friendly micro-flora and *Candida* is disturbed and causes an overgrowth of malignant yeast in the gastrointestinal tract. This balance can be disturbed by over-prescription of antibiotics (that don't discriminate between bad bacteria and friendly bacteria), over-consumption of sugar and dairy (according to July 1984 issue of the *Journal of Reproductive Medicine*), and bad food combining, which results in undigested food traveling down the gastrointestinal tract. Chronic *candidiasis* has been clinically proven to cause a wide variety of symptoms in virtually every system of the body. Most people suffering from *candidiasis* rarely suspect it as the cause of their ill health. The symptoms are so numerous and seemingly unrelated that medical doctors usually just treat the consequential complications (such as fatigue, arthritis, depression, migraine, etc.) and never seek the underlying cause.

When Should You Drink?

The answer—drink lots of liquids about half an hour before you eat and then again an hour after you eat. In addition, supplement your meal with vegetables rich in liquids, which will provide the necessary lubrication you need with your food. Try this a few times and see how much lighter you feel after a meal.

While we're on the subject of water, drink lots of it throughout the day. Almost every chemical process that happens in your body requires water. In addition, you need water to flush out toxins and excess fat. It is recommended to drink about eight cups of purified or spring water throughout the day. Sodas, juices, and coffee don't count.

In summary, be aware of what you put on your plate and what kind of combinations you ask your stomach to deal with. If you're asking your stomach to deal with the diet of a lion, cow, ape, and pig all at the same time, don't be surprised if your stomach comes back at you with a vengeance, in the form of heartburn, acid reflux, or other ailments.

Getting in the Habit

Here's an exercise to help you get in the habit of properly combining the different food groups.

For the next week observe what you eat for lunch. Is it a sandwich? Meat with potatoes or rice? Whatever the combo might be, pay attention and if you notice you're making poor combination choices, try some substitutes.

For example, if you're used to eating chicken and rice, try to replace the rice with raw or steamed vegetables. If it's a sandwich (bread is a carbohydrate), try and have it only with vegetables.

You might also try some brown rice or whole wheat pasta (carbohydrates) with vegetables or beans; it's a great source of complex carbohydrates and light protein.

Finally, pay attention to your drinking habits (and I don't mean you should join AA!). If you typically drink soda or fruit juice with your meal, try and avoid drinking any liquids for half hour before you eat to an hour afterwards. Notice how it makes you feel. If you absolutely have to have some liquids, have a glass of red wine or beer with your meal. These are fermented and will not impair digestion.

Becoming mindful about your food combinations will make a big difference to how you feel after a meal, as well as your overall sense of well-being.

Chapter 4

Exercise & Breathing: The Ultimate Maintenance Program

If we could give every individual the right amount of
nourishment and exercise, not too little and not too
much, we would have found the safest way to health.
—Hippocrates

Exercise is a tune-up for our body. Without regular exercise our blood becomes stagnant, cells starve for lack of a proper oxygen supply, and toxins are not eliminated properly from peripheral tissue and the blood stream. On top of that, we won't burn all the energy we receive from our food, which means we gain weight and put ourselves at risk of heart disease and diabetes.

Our heart is a muscle, and as with any muscle it needs some workout. When we don't exercise enough our heart becomes weak and a weak heart clearly leads to ... trouble.

Studies have shown that men who are physically active on a regular basis have a lower overall mortality rate than those who are physically inactive (and the same is presumed for women on the basis of extrapolation). Exercise appears to be especially effective in improving health status in six disease-specific areas: heart disease, hypertension, obesity, diabetes, osteoporosis, and diminished psychological well-being.

Exercise is also instrumental for proper function of the lymphatic system. The lymphatic system returns excess interstitial fluid to the blood, hence maintaining proper blood pressure and preventing edema (swelling), absorbs fats and fat-soluble vitamins, and probably its most-known function—providing defense against invaders and disease.

Unlike the cardiovascular system, which relies on the heart for circulation, the lymphatic system doesn't have a pump to initiate circulation. Instead, it relies on body movements to initiate circulation. If you are accustomed to a sedentary lifestyle, chances are your lymphatic system will become stagnant and as a result your immune system as well as fat elimination will be compromised.

You see, as human beings we were designed to move. Our ancestors used to be in constant movement, whether gathering plants and roots or when chasing after animals for meat. Even when humans settled in agricultural communities they were still in constant movement, plowing and harvesting their fields or shepherding their herds. Physiologically you are not any different than your ancestors and so you should strive to move as much as possible throughout the day.

Imagine someone waking you in the middle of the night, shoving bacon and eggs in your mouth, and telling you, "Eat!" That's exactly what you're asking of your digestive system if you eat breakfast without any prior physical activity. Exercising first thing in the morning, before breakfast, every day for only ten or fifteen minutes is highly beneficial as it kicks your metabolism into action and wakes up the digestive organs. As a result your body will burn fats and sugars more effectively throughout the day. This will mean an increase in energy levels and stamina and a decrease in waistline and body-fat percentage.

Simple Ways to Exercise

Walking

Walking is the easiest and safest way to adopt an exercise regimen. It doesn't require a membership or any special equipment—just a pair of sneakers. When weather permits, walking in nature is highly encouraged. When it rains the mall will do just fine.

You can also adopt a walking buddy for support and accountability. If you don't show up, your buddy will give you a piece of his/her mind.

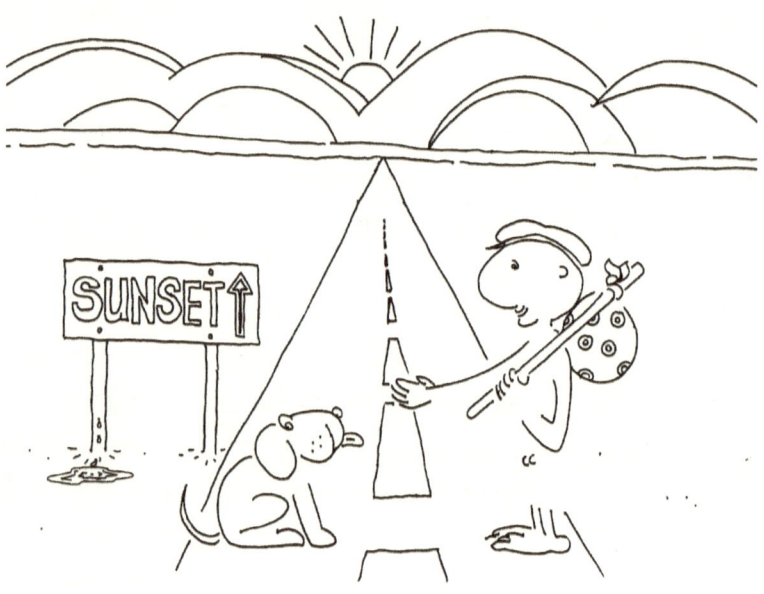

Joe: *Would you like to be my walking buddy?*

Rusty: *As long as I can pee wherever I want!*

Running

About 1.2 million years ago humans shed their hair[7] and developed four times the number of sweat glands of other mammals. Some evolutionary theories suggest these changes allowed early humans to stay

---

[7]   Rogers AR, Iltis D, & Wooding S, 2004. Genetic variation at the MC1R locus and the time since loss of human body hair. *Current Anthropology, 45*(1): 105–108.

cool while they outran and exhausted the other animals, who overheated in contrast. This development pushed humans to the top of the food chain. My conclusion: humans were born to run!

Running doesn't require complex equipment or membership in most cases. Running is also one of the best ways to lose weight. The up and down motion of running actually exercises *every cell* in your body—even down to your fingernails! This causes the cells to burn more energy, which in turn leads to weight loss. Think about it, have you ever seen an overweight runner?

You should be careful, though; running can hurt your joints and spine. If you choose to run for exercise, make sure you listen to your body.

Swimming

Swimming is an excellent form of exercise that works all the major muscle groups, as well as the lungs and heart. If you're lucky enough to live by the ocean or a lake then you'll have the pleasure of swimming in a health club called Nature. But a word of advice; make sure you learn how to swim before trying this invigorating form of exercise.

Weight Lifting and Weight Bearing

Weightlifting is also an excellent way to stimulate muscle growth and strengthen bones. It also helps in preventing osteoporosis as you age. However, unless you have equipment at home, a gym membership will be required. It is also advisable to hook up with a trainer before commencing this type of workout.

> What is the difference between weight lifting and weight bearing? Weight bearing exercises are exercises that utilize the body's own weight. In a way walking and standing are weight bearing, as they bear the weight of the body. Other weight-bearing exercises include balancing poses, sit-ups, and pushups, just to name a few. Swimming doesn't count as weight bearing as the body is submerged in water. Weight-bearing exercises are extremely important for maintaining bone density and preventing osteoporosis in later years.

Yoga

Yoga is a great form of exercise that helps balance the body, mind, and soul. The different yoga postures help to both stretch and strengthen the muscles, tissue, and bones. Yoga also increases blood flow to remote tissues, thereby internally cleansing and detoxifying your body. Although it's highly recommended to learn yoga with a certified instructor, after a few lessons it can be done privately in the comfort of your own home.

Many folks hesitate to try yoga because they fear they are not flexible enough. That's like not wanting to learn how to drive because … you don't know how to drive. Yoga is not a race. All you have to do is get started. So what are you waiting for?

Tai Chi

In Chinese the word chi (qi) represents the internal energetic life force we all possess. Tai Chi is a form of martial arts that is intended to increase this vital life force. Tai Chi consists of series of rhythmic movements. It is very safe and not physically challenging, which makes it an ideal exercise for older people. Much like yoga, Tai Chi should first be learned from a certified instructor before continuing on your own. Don't get yourself confused with the *Karate Kid,* though—that's a whole different movie.

Breathing

Breathing is the most basic and essential part of our lives. It is more important than food or water. If we stop breathing for just over five minutes we cease to exist. However, most of us take breathing for granted and even more crucially, do not even pay attention to the way we breathe. And most of us also breathe incorrectly by expanding our lungs. The proper way to breathe is by expanding your diaphragm. This method allows more air to enter your lungs and in addition calms and relaxes the nervous system.

The following is a breathing technique I recommend you perform every morning. It's called the *Skull Shining* technique, as it makes the skull shine. It strengthens the diaphragm, helps release toxins from the lungs, and most importantly, strengthens the immune system:

1. Sit comfortably in a chair with a straight back.

2. Close your eyes and take a deep inhalation through your nose by expanding your diaphragm.

3. Exhale completely through your nose and push your belly as if you're trying to touch your back with your belly.

4. Breathe in and allow your diaphragm to expand again.

5. Now exhale while vigorously pushing your diaphragm toward your back.

6. Allow your diaphragm to naturally expand again.

7. With quick motions repeat this process of vigorously exhaling and naturally allowing the diaphragm to expand.

8. Ultimately you should be able to commence three sets of thirty-six exhalations, always inhaling and exhaling through your nose.

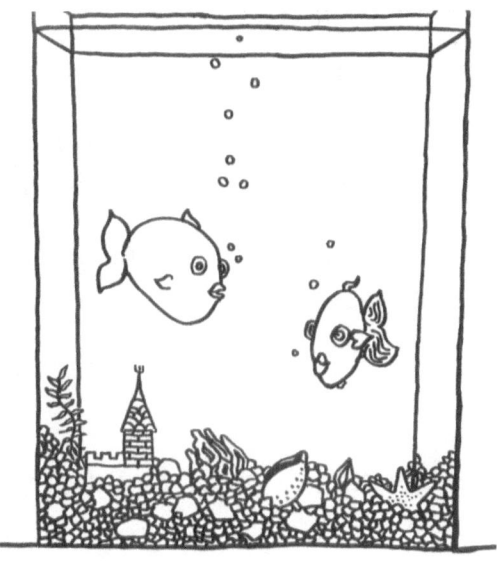

A. *Did you do the Skull Shining breathing exercise this morning?*

B. *No*

A. *Why not?*

B. *My wife says I make too many bubbles ...*

Getting in the habit:

The following is an exercise to get you in the habit of… exercising (if you don't already do so):

Next week (not the following one or the one after):

1. Get yourself a pair of walking sneakers (if you don't already have them).

2. Find a place where you will enjoy walking. This can be a park, a nature reserve nearby, or

even your own neighborhood, as long as it's easily accessible.

3. Mark three days on the calendar in which you'll commit to walking at least twenty minutes.

4. Mark the actual time for each day that you commit to walk.

5. Find a walking buddy to accompany you (optional).

6. Forget about any other commitments during your walking time and walk for at least twenty minutes.

7. Repeat the above steps the following week and the one after. Try to slowly increase the duration, intensity, and the amount of days you walk.

In wintertime, make a commitment to join a gym where you feel comfortable.

After joining, sign up with a personal trainer, at least for the first month. A personal trainer will keep you accountable and in addition teach you how to properly use all equipment. He or she will set up a workout regimen for you, which you can later continue on your own.

If you commit to this program, I promise you will feel a tremendous improvement in your well-being, both physically and mentally.

Chapter 5

Detox: The Most Important Thing You Can Do for Your Health

Self-love, my liege, is not so vile a sin, as self-neglecting.
—William Shakespeare

We all take a shower at least once a day (at least I hope we do!). It is just as important to clean our internal organs once in a while. Can you imagine what your home would look like if your drains got clogged? Well, the sewer would soon flood and a bad odor and pests would follow.

The intestines and colon are our drain system. The Royal Academy of Physicians of Great Britain estimates that 90 percent of all disease and discomfort is directly, or indirectly, related to an unclean colon.[8]

---

[8]   *Global College of Natural Medicine Study Guide.* Toxicity & Detoxi-
       fication, Santa Cruz, California: GCNM, 2004–2005

When we eat, the essential nutrients are absorbed into the blood stream through the intestinal walls. The rest keeps moving down the intestines and through the colon to be eliminated. However, since most of us eat a diet that is rich in animal food and low in fiber, some of these food residues accumulate on the intestinal and colon wall. Over time there is a buildup.

The results of this residue buildup are twofold. On the one hand, it blocks essential nutrients from entering the blood stream, leaving us fatigued and improperly nourished. On the other hand, it acts as a breeding ground for bacteria, viruses, fungi, and other parasitic hosts who continuously contaminate our blood stream, jeopardizing our immune system. *This process can be one of the major reasons for a variety of different ailments and allergies,* from a simple flu to asthma and even cancer.

> The colon hosts nearly sixty varieties of microflora or bacteria. Their role is to aid in the breakdown and digestion of vital nutrients, help maintain proper PH (acidic-alkaline) balance, and prevent propagation of harmful bacteria. These microflora also provide important functions such as the synthesis of folic acid and other valuable nutrients from food, including vitamin K and portions of the B complex. *Bacillus coli* and *acidophilus* comprise the majority of healthy bacteria in the colon along with other disease-producing bacteria in lesser numbers. In a healthy colon the beneficial bacteria outnumber the harmful bacteria.

Trouble begins when as a result of exposure to elements such as toxic food and antibiotics, this delicate balance is compromised.

It is crucial, then, to detoxify our colon at least twice a year. And the best time is during the traditional cleaning seasons, spring and autumn. A good colon detoxifying product should include ingredients to restore flora and bacterial and PH balance in the colon.

Detoxifying Other Organs

In addition to the colon and intestines, it is also important to cleanse and detoxify the rest of our internal organs of all the toxins that accumulate over time. Make sure you also clean the liver and kidneys. Both these organs are responsible for the removal of toxins from the digestive system and blood respectively. If they are clogged they can't do their job properly, which means there are more toxins circulating in your bloodstream. The lungs and skin are two other organs that can benefit immensely from periodic cleansing, and some detoxification products are aimed at cleansing these vital organs.

There are many cleansing programs and products out there. Some last ten days and some are for thirty or ninety days. Some are more general and some more focused. They range in price from $17 to about $150. I recommend you start with a simple ten-day program and try a different one every few months until you find the one that is right for you. Start with a colon cleanse, and when you're done, move on to the liver and finally the kidneys.

Colonic irrigation is a subject that brings some bad connotations to most people's minds. However, if you consider that the average American may be carrying as much as ten to twenty-five pounds of impacted fecal matter in his/her colon and that most diseases begin in the colon, you may see the benefit of incorporating colon irrigation into your detoxification program. With the right equipment, colonic irrigation can be administered at home; all you need is a special shower head that has the ability to have a hose connected to it. (It can be purchased at Home Depot for about $35.) In order to perform the irrigation, lie in your bath tub and place the end of the hose against the anus. Do not insert the hose! Next, allow for the flow of warm water to travel up your colon by means of pressure. You will know when it's time to stop and hop onto the toilet. You may repeat this process a few times until the water coming out of you is clean. If you're concerned about performing colonic irrigation on your own, there are many clinics that specialize in it. I urge you to try it. It might sound bad at first, but you will feel so energetic and light afterwards you might think you are flying.

As I was writing these lines, the subject of detoxification came up on a few morning shows and in most of them experts seemed to think detoxification wasn't a good idea. Their argument was that fasting for ten days and drinking nothing but lemon juice with cayenne pepper (Master Cleanse) can lead to loss of muscle tone and jeopardize the immune system. I must partially agree with them; I think that these kinds of extreme detoxification methods should be practiced only by people who have previous experience with prolonged fasting and should be done in a state of rest, under supervision, in a retreat, for example. However, I don't think this contradicts the use of colon cleanse products, or even should you decide to fast for one day drinking nothing but citrus (orange or grapefruit) juice, which can be extremely beneficial to your digestive system.

Sam's Story:

Sam was diagnosed by a medical doctor with Folliculitis; an infection of the hair follicles on his head and face. The medical doctor, who examined Sam for less than fifteen minutes, determined that the only way to treat this condition is with oral antibiotic treatment *for life!*

Needless to say, Sam was not too thrilled about taking antibiotics on a regular basis for the rest of his life and so he was seeking an alternative treatment when he got to me.

Upon interviewing Sam two things became rather apparent; Sam used to eat a diet that at times consisted of high amounts of animal-based protein and fat, and

Sam loved to drink a bottle of beer every day after work. Being of Italian origin he also loved pasta.

The first thing I recommended to Sam was to undergo a detoxification program, as it seemed that the animal fat and protein rich diet may have contributed to high levels of toxins in his digestive tract and blood. These toxins may have translated to infection of the hair follicles.

My second recommendation was to try and avoid beer and other wheat products such as pasta as much as possible. The reason is that some people develop sensitivities to certain types of food, which can turn into different imbalances, and the tell-tale sign is usually when an individual loves a certain type of food almost to the point of addiction. Wheat is a very common such food.

After a ten-day intestinal detoxification program and avoiding any wheat products as much as possible, Sam's condition improved dramatically, and within a period of one month there seem to have been no additional irruptions or worsening of his condition. At the time of writing, Sam has yet to undergo liver, kidneys and blood detoxification programs.

Furthermore, Sam is reporting that severe back aches he used to suffer have also disappeared. This can be attributed to the elimination of wheat products, as wheat is known in the nutrition world to cause back pain.

I will summarize In Sam's own words; "I decided to swap an addiction to beer, meat and pasta with the addiction to *feeling clean.*"

Getting in the Habit

Since most people don't get enough fiber, which helps keep their colon clean, chances are you don't either.

What I suggest is that the next time you go shopping, stop by the oatmeal/cereal section and pick up a box of instant oatmeal, or better yet, raw oats.

For the next week, try and incorporate either instant oatmeal (just add hot water and it's ready) or raw oatmeal (rolled oats) into your breakfast.

My favorite breakfast is raw oatmeal with raw sunflower seeds, pecans, sliced almonds, and organic strawberries (in season) or organic cranberry mix in rice milk. This is the kind of breakfast that provides you with a host of essential nutrients, as well as an adequate supply of dietary fiber. (Just make sure you leave yourself enough time to visit the bathroom—you'll need it!)

When you make a commitment to detoxify your internal organs you'll quickly start to feel what it's like to be clean on the inside, light, alert, and full of energy.

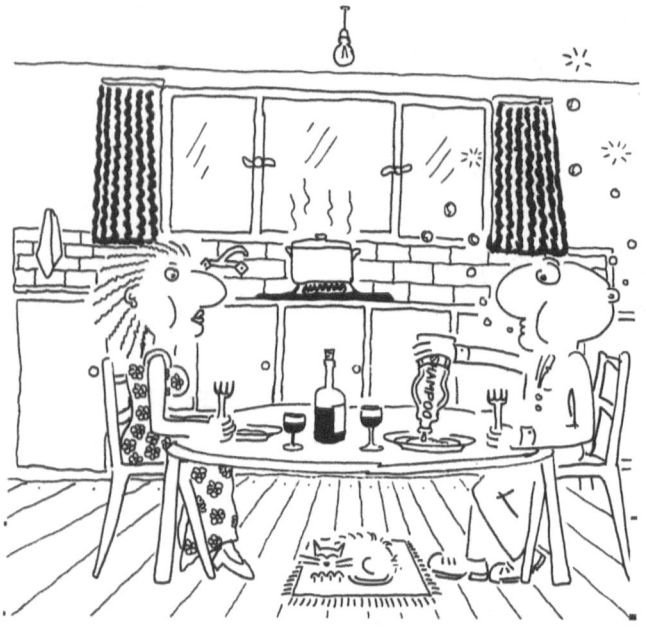

Wife: *What on earth are you doing?*

Husband: *Swallowing soap.*

Wife: *Why ... ?*

Husband: *The book said it's important to clean on the inside. You should try it too my dear ...*

Chapter 6

To Dairy or Not to Dairy, That is the Question

*Humans are the only mammal weaned off its mum
only to spend the rest of its life stuck under the
udders of a completely different species.
—Phillip Day, author of* Health Wars

Here are some points to consider in regard to milk; we are the only mammal that continues to consume milk after adulthood. We are also the only mammal that consumes another mammal's milk voluntarily (and that makes the cow go "duh" instead of "moo"). The cows, whose milk we drink, are supposed to feed on grass in open pastures but in many cases end up eating farm feed made up of stale bakery waste and even leftover parts from meat-processing facilities. They are also injected with hormones and antibiotics that enter our system once we consume their milk.

This jeopardizes our own immune system, putting us at risk for different kinds of cancer.

Milk and Pasteurization

In today's Western society we have come to believe that milk and other dairy products are essential for our growth and well-being. Although that might hold water if you are blood type B and consuming organic, non-pasteurized dairy products, those kinds of products are extremely hard, if not impossible, to find in today's supermarkets. Pasteurization is used in order to kill any bacteria or germs that exist in the milk and prolong its shelf-life. However, this same process also eliminates all the vital amino acids, enzymes, and nutrients that are essential for digesting milk and making it beneficial for our bodies. Pasteurization leaves the milk impotent and utterly empty of nutrients. Furthermore, because of the lack of enzymes and nutrients, the milk actually becomes toxic to us and may increase the burden on our elimination system.

According to Dr. Peter J. D'Adamo author of *Eat Right for Your Type,* blood type B developed in humans around 15,000–10,000 BC in the Himalaya region of today's Pakistan and India, when early humans migrated from the warm savannas of Africa to the dry, cold climate of the Himalayas and probably as a reaction to this change in climate. Blood type B developed first among

Mongolian and Caucasian mixed tribes. As these tribes spread along Asia, southeast Asia, and later Eastern and northern Europe, they also spread their blood type along with their culture, which depended on raising animals and herding. Their herds provided them with both meat and milk, and so they adapted to consumption of milk. Indeed, to this day people with blood type B, who are predominant in Eastern Europe and Asia, can tolerate dairy better than other blood types.

In a ten-year study, conducted in the 1930s by Dr. Francis M. Pottenger Jr. on the relative effects of a diet containing only processed food including pasteurized milk and a diet containing only raw food including raw milk on nine hundred cats, two groups of cats were fed only raw food and raw non-pasteurized milk and the other three groups only processed food and pasteurized milk. The findings were interesting; the raw food, raw milk group grew healthier and stronger with good bone density, wide palates with plenty of space for teeth, shiny fur no parasites, or disease and reproductive ease, resulting in plenty of offspring.

In contrast the processed food, pasteurized milk groups developed host of degenerative health conditions toward the end of their life; arthritis, allergies, diabetes, hypothyroidism, personality changes, osteoporosis, and many other degenerative diseases encountered by human medicine. Those health conditions continued with the second generation, although they appeared earlier; towards the middle of their life span and in the third generation they appeared early in their life. As to the fourth generation—there was none! That might help explain the alarming rates of infertility in our society today, not to mention the above degenerative health conditions many elderly people in the Western world suffer from.

In the book *Healthy to 100* authors Alexa Fleckenstein MD and Rose Weisman describe some of the risks associated with dairy consumption:

- Milk is a high-caloric liquid that is contributing heavily (pun intended) to our present epidemic of overweight population.

- Dairy adds more protein to our already too protein-rich fare. The extra protein is digested and broken down to acidic purines, which need buffering before they can be expelled from the body. *Your body takes the alkaline calcium from your bones to buffer the acidic purines, thus promoting bone loss.*

- Dairy is mucus-producing food, bad for asthma, bronchitis, and hay fever.

- Dairy promotes inflammation in your body, thus creating and exacerbating arthritis, bursitis, tendonitis, heart disease, diabetes, and cancer (among others).

The Alternatives

So now we have two questions; what can I substitute for cows' milk, and where can I find an alternate source of calcium if I drop dairy products? Although it's still a processed product, soy milk is a great alternative. Some folks complain that they don't like the taste of soymilk. To that I say, try it for fourteen days, after which I promise you will never consume cows' milk again. Other excellent alternatives are almond or rice or oat milk, which are even better for you than soy.

Mother Nature has the answer to the second question; calcium is abundant in broccoli, cabbage and green leafy vegetables as well as in nuts, especially almonds and sesame seeds. Asparagus, soy products, salmon, and sardines all contain high levels of calcium.

The bottom line: replace dairy products with those listed above and you are sure to notice the difference in your well-being.

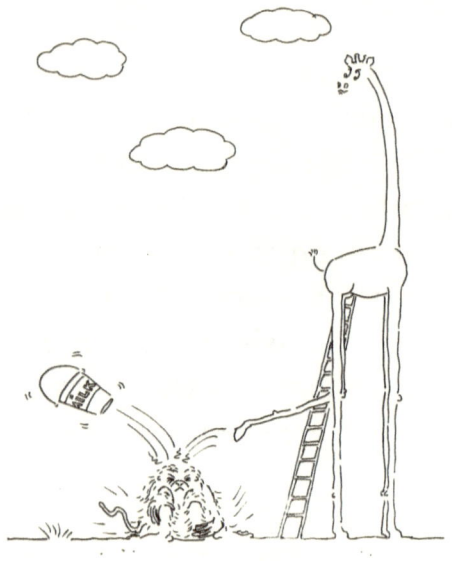

Monkey: *Hey Giraffe, mind if I get some of your milk?*

Giraffe: *Get the ... out of here!*

Getting in the Habit

The next time you visit the supermarket, purchase some rice, nuts, or soy milk. For the next week substitute one of the above milks for dairy milk in your coffee and with your cereal. It might not taste good in the beginning, but since you are on a mission to adopt a healthier life style, *you can do it!*

By the end of this week your taste buds should be used to the taste of alternative milk. If not, try it for one more week. Many people have been able to make this shift, and so can you. The contribution to your health and sense of well-being will be enormous.

Chapter 7

Fats: The Good and the Bad

Most people in the Western world eat too much
saturated fat, the kind that kills, and too little
of the essential fats, the kind that heal.
—Patrick Holford,
head of The Institute for Optimum Nutrition

Fats have gotten a bad rap in recent years. From low-fat foods to low-fat diets, we do everything we can to avoid any kind of fat, sometimes with the result that we eat more sugar. However, not all fats are bad for us. If they were, how can we explain the fat-rich diet of the Inuit people (Eskimos) who boast extremely low incidences of heart disease? The answer is that while some fats are bad for us, some are actually beneficial and instrumental to our health.

In his book *The Tao of Health, Sex & Longevity,* author Daniel P. Reid explains the benefits of the Eskimo diet: "Eskimos who traditionally ate a diet that consisted almost entirely of raw meat, raw fat and raw fish, had never been known to suffer arthritis, heart disease or any other chronic ailment until they started eating the packaged processed foods introduced to them by their *'civilized'* brethren from America. The Eskimos were the only tribe in all of North and South America that never developed the tradition of a tribal 'medicine man' because they virtually never got sick. Indeed the word 'Eskimo' comes from an old Indian term which means 'he who eats it raw,' and therein lies the secret of their former health and longevity."

The Bad

The fats that are dangerous to our health are saturated and trans fats. These are the kind you find in potato chips, deep-fried foods, margarine, and refined vegetable oils such as corn or sunflower oils. These types of fats are actually toxic to our system and can result in obesity or even heart disease and cancer. It's imperative to cut these kinds of fats out of your diet as much as possible, especially if you'd like to reach old age full of vim and vigor.

The Good

Fats that are beneficial to our health are Omega 6 and Omega 3 essential fatty acids (EFA). These fats are now the celebrities of the nutrition world and studies have shown that they contribute to a healthy brain, help reduce inflammation, stabilize blood sugar levels, and help prevent coronary heart disease. Generally we should consume both Omega 3 and 6 in equal amounts.

So where can I find these essential fats, you must be asking? Omega 3 fatty acids are harder to obtain in modern diets since they are pronged to damage from cooking. Omega 3 fatty acids are derived from alpha-linolenic acid, which is metabolized into EPA (eicosapentaenoic acid) that then turns to DHA (docosahexaenoic acid). The building blocks of omega 3 fatty acids are prevalent in cold-water fish such as mackerel, herring, salmon, sardines, and lake trout. It's also prevalent in green leafy vegetables as well as the following nuts and seeds: flax, hemp, pumpkin, and walnut.

The building blocks for omega 6, a byproduct of linoleic acid, which is converted by the body into gamma-linolenic acid (GLA), are common in sunflower seeds, pumpkin seeds, safflower seeds, sesame, corn, walnuts, and soybeans and especially hemp (it might not be healthy to smoke but it's sure healthy to eat). It's best to consume all these nuts and seeds raw and unsalted as the process of roasting and heating ruins these essential fats. And the richest sources of GLA are evening primrose oil and borage oil. Since these oils are already in GLA form, if you use them in supplement form, you will need less overall oil to obtain enough Omega 6 fats.

> Patrick Holford, head of the Optimum Nutrition Institute in the UK and author of *The New Optimum Nutrition Bible* describes the increasingly complex process in which omega 3 fatty acids are formed as we move up the food chain: "Plankton for example, the staple food of small fish, is rich in alpha-linolenic acid. The little fish eat the plankton, then the carnivorous fish, like mackerel or herring, eat the small fish, which have converted some of their alpha-linolenic acid into more complex fats. The carnivorous fish continue the conversion. Seals eat them and have the highest EPA and DHA concentration. Finally, Eskimos eat the seals and benefit from a ready-made meal of EPA and DHA. You, if you want to have a healthy brain and body … eat Eskimos!"

The Mediterranean Way

Another great oil is olive oil. Although olive oil doesn't contain EFAs (essential fatty acids), it does contain a small amount of phytochemicals (do not attempt to pronounce this word), which results in fewer trans fats being consumed. In addition, olive oil is cold pressed, which makes it much safer than refined vegetable oils such as sunflower oil. Finally, if for some reason you ever decide to fry your food, olive oil should be the oil of choice. Besides tasting better, it also oxidizes slower than other oils when exposed to heat, which means less free radicals in your body (and I'm not talking about freedom fighters here). It's better for your mouth and better for your health. And that my friends, is a home run.

Oxidation is defined as the interaction between *oxygen* molecules and all the different substances they may contact, from metal to living tissue. Technically, however, with the discovery of electrons, oxidation came to be more precisely defined as the loss of at least one *electron* when two or more substances interact.

Oxygen is the basis of all plant and animal life. It is the most important nutrient needed by every cell, every second of the day. But through biochemical reactions, oxygen can become unstable when individual oxygen molecules become separated (known as free radicals) and *oxidize* cells, meaning to rob them of their electrons, leaving the molecules of these cells unstable. This can lead to cell damage that triggers inflammation, arterial damage, aging, and even cancer.

Getting in the Habit

Here's a tip for getting enough essential fatty acids in your diet: add a handful of sunflower seeds, hemp seeds, and walnuts to your morning cereal. They won't just make the cereal healthier but also tastier. If cereal is not a part of your morning routine, you can keep a box of mixed organic raw nuts in your car for a healthy, satisfying snack on your way to and from work.

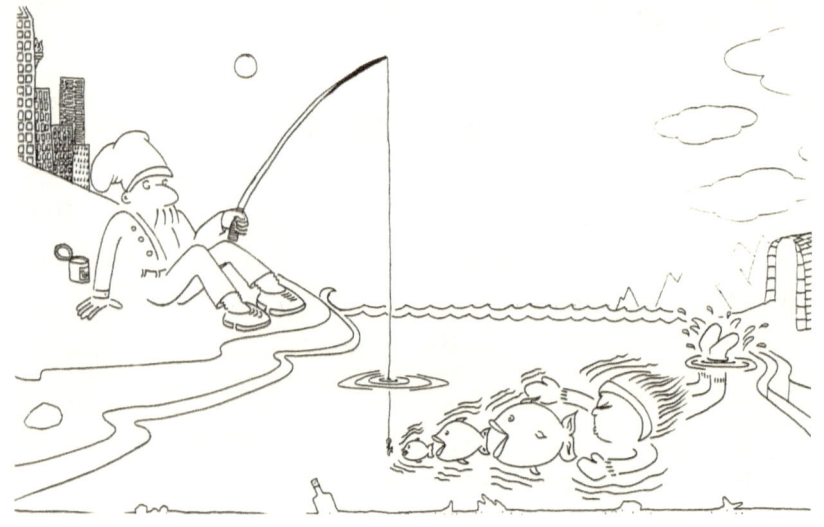

The best way to fish for Eskimos

Chapter 8

Supplementing for Life

Vitamins, minerals and other supplements won't compensate for a poor diet, but they can help fill nutritional gaps in a good one.
—*Dr. Andrew Weil*

It's very hard to receive all the nutrients we need from food alone, especially if we're eating the over-processed, commercial produce so prevalent in our supermarkets and grocery stores. Our bodies need the right vitamins and minerals in order to function to their maximum efficiency. We also need a group of nutrients called anti-oxidants to enhance and support our immune system.

The only way to ensure that we're adequately receiving all these nutrients is by supplementing with vitamins, minerals, and vital herbs.

Using supplements is like fertilizing your lawn. You don't know you need it until there are signs of trouble. For this reason I recommend using certain basic supplements as a preventive policy against major nutrient deficiencies. You could call it umbrella insurance! Later on you can add to this basic formula depending on your nutritional needs, lifestyle, and physical and mental activities.

Please remember, though, supplementing is not a substitute for a balanced, healthy diet. It is what its name suggests: a supplement to an otherwise healthy lifestyle.

I recommend the following on a daily basis:

- A good multi-vitamin that provides a broad spectrum of vitamins and minerals. One that I personally like and use is Every Man by New Chapter* (they also have Every Woman).

- Vitamin C is extremely important for many of the body's functions. It strengthens the immune system, fights infections, keeps bones, skin, and joints firm and strong, detoxifies pollutants, and protects against cancer and heart disease. It also helps make anti-stress hormones and turns food into energy. It should have been called vitamin S(uper)!

  The best is vitamin C with bioflavonoid or Ester C.

Supplementary range: 800 to 2800mg daily

- Vitamin E is an extremely important anti-oxidant that guards against free radicals and protects the cells from damage, including cancer. Vitamin E also prevents blood clots, improves wound healing and fertility, and is good for the skin *(and that, ladies, is worth its price in gold)!*

Supplementary range: 225 to 800 IU daily.

- B Vitamins are extremely important but are usually present in sufficient amounts in a good multi-vitamin. However, for those who are nursing, expecting, or even thinking about trying to get pregnant, I recommend supplementing with folic acid. Folic acid is extremely important for the fetus and newborn's brain development.

Supplementary range (for folic acid): 200 to 600 mcg daily.

- Vitamin B12 is an essential for vegetarians. Typically our only sources for Vitamin B12 are meat and fish. Therefore, it's extremely important for vegetarians to supplement with this important B Vitamin.

- Omega 3: we discussed the importance of Omega 3 Fatty Acids in the chapter about fats. Omega 3 promotes a healthy heart, thins the blood, helps to reduce inflammation, improves functioning of the nervous system, and relieves depression, schizophrenia, ADD, hyperactivity, and autism. It also improves sleep and skin conditions, helps balance hormones, and reduces insulin resistance. By God, is there anything Omega 3 doesn't do? This thing is like kryptonite.

Supplementary range: EPA 150 to 550 mg DHA 100 to 500 mg

- A good anti-oxidant blend: anti-oxidants are important to use as protection against cell degeneration, cancer, and other disease. The one that I use is Supercritical Antioxidants by New Chapter* and contains turmeric, green tea, cloves, ginger, parsley, peppermint, and rosemary.

The following are optional supplements with great benefits:

- Turmeric: an important anti-oxidant in itself, studies have shown that turmeric helps to significantly reduce inflammation and can reduce, and even prevent, the growth of cancer cells. I highly recommend it for those who suffer from arthritis.

- Garlic: another important anti-oxidant that can enhance immunity, help prevent cancer, and reduce cholesterol and high blood pressure.

- Probiotics blend (acidophilus and bifidus): the friendly bacteria that inhabit our colon and help in the breakdown of food are exposed to daily attacks from parasites, fungi, and antibiotics. It's essential to replenish these friendly bacteria in order to keep yeast infections and parasites at bay.

- CoQ10: a supplement that increases oxygen utilization on a cellular level (especially in the heart) and aerobic capacity. Highly recommended for athletes and those who suffer from heart disease.

- Green Tea (in liquid form): green tea is an anti-oxidant in its own right. However, the reason I recommend it is for its enzymatic activity.[9] People in Asia drink green tea at the end of a meal. The reason? It assists in proper digestion due to its rich enzymatic activity. I recommend drinking green tea every day after dinner (decaffeinated if you have sleeping problems). This will help your digestive system to do its work more effectively.

- Gingko, ginseng, and Goto Kola all improve circulation, concentration, and stamina. Choose

---

[9] *Nutrition*, Volume 23, Issue 9, 687–95

the one that is right for you, as they all have different attributes. Ladies, I'll let you in on a little secret—ginseng helps … well, put it this way, the Chinese use it a lot and there are now more than one billion Chinese people.

- Echinacea: a natural antibiotic; take with the first signs of cold or flu.

* I am not affiliated in any way with New Chapter. I simply find their products of high quality and use them myself.

Danny's Story: when Danny came to see me he was suffering from an excruciating pain in his right shoulder and didn't wish to continue with pain relievers such as Ibuprofen, which were prescribed to him. In addition to some dietary changes, I also recommended to Danny to try supplemental turmeric, as turmeric has been scientifically proven to help reduce inflammation. A couple of days later I received an ecstatic phone call from Danny; not only his pain was completely gone and he was pain free for the first time in many, many months, but in addition, a nagging gingivitis he was suffering from also disappeared. It's no surprise Turmeric is regarded as the "Wonder Herb".

Getting in the Habit

This week find a local health store. Make some time to go in and familiarize yourself with the supplements

I've detailed above. Depending on your budget, pick out a few and start using them on a daily basis. Most supplements absorb better when taken with food. Pay attention to how they make you feel. The next week repeat this process with more supplements if needed.

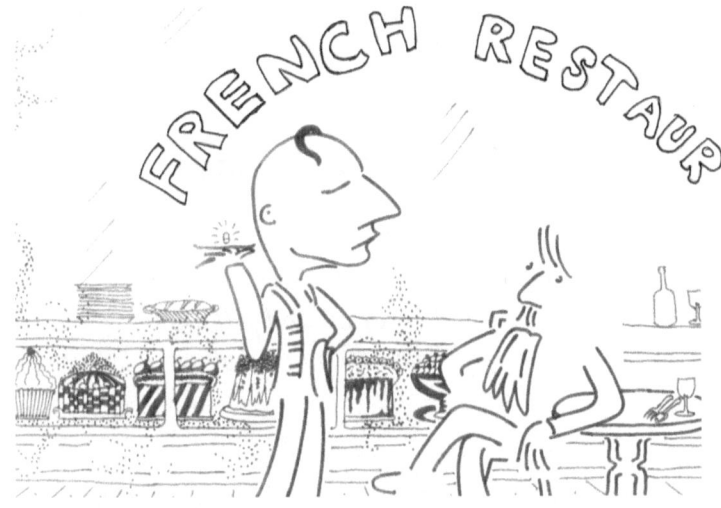

*"Here you go, sir, vitamin C in vitamin
A reduction. Enjoy your meal!"*

Chapter 9

It's All in the Elimination

The underlying basis of Natural Hygiene is that the body is self-cleansing, self-healing and self maintaining.
—*Harvey Diamond, #1 best-selling co-author of* Fit for Life

It goes without saying: *no late night meals or snacks!* Still, while most people are aware that eating before bedtime is counterproductive to losing weight or maintaining a healthy body, they persist in the habit.

Here are some facts that may help you stay away from the fridge when Jay Leno or David Letterman are on. Our bodies have a tremendous healing power, and every night around 8:00 to 9:00 PM our digestive tract goes into assimilation and detoxification mode. This is the time that the food we've eaten all day is assimilated by our intestines. They squeeze out all of the nutrients overnight while our body puts the nutrients to work, replenishing cells and rejuvenating and ridding itself of any toxins, including excess fat.

If we eat after 8 PM the digestive system is still busy breaking down the food we just ate and cannot kick into assimilation and detoxification mode. Once we lie down, gravity also works against our digestive system and the food we ate late gets stuck in our gut overnight, to rot and ferment. If we eat less than three hours before going to sleep on a regular basis, our body is consistently trying to digest food when it's really time to assimilate and detoxify. This just makes it that much harder for us to get rid of toxins and excess fat.

Many dietitians and nutritionists today advise their clients to eat five to six small meals a day, also known as grazing. Grazing, though, is practiced in nature by herbivorous animals (plant eating), and humans are primarily omnivorous (eating both plants and animals). According to John Douillard, author of *The 3- Season Diet,* when we graze our body is constantly busy breaking down and metabolizing sugars from the food we just ate. Sugars or carbohydrates are good source of energy for *flight or fight* situations, as it can rapidly be absorbed by the body to supply a quick surge of energy. But as you learned before (chapter 2), it can also lead to a rollercoaster effect in which you are constantly craving more food.

On the other hand, when you resort to eating three fulfilling meals a day, breakfast before 9:00 AM, lunch between 10:00 AM and 2:00 PM when metabolism is in its peak, and a light dinner between 5:00 and 7:00 PM with no snacks whatsoever in between, you allow your digestive system to first break sugars, but once the body finished metabolizing sugar, it will switch to burning fat for energy. This process has a few benefits. Fat provides a more stable and sustainable form of energy than sugar. It stabilizes blood sugar levels and reduces cravings. Finally, as you burn more fat instead of sugar you are likely to lose excess fat and reach your optimal weight. When you adopt this kind of meal schedule, you will find it is much easier to refrain from late meals or snacks and actually fast while burning fat and resting your digestive system from 7:00 PM to 7:00 AM.

Also, when we eat before going to sleep, we don't burn the energy we just put into our body. Since this energy cannot be used, it has to be stored somewhere. And yes, you guessed it, it all goes into the "storage room" of our body—the fat tissue, a sure way to gain more fat.

The bottom line: after 8:00 PM watch TV, play with your kids, or just relax. Whatever you do, stay away from the fridge.

Getting in the Habit

For the next week pay attention to the time you eat dinner. If you eat dinner after 8:00 PM on a consistent basis, make a conscious effort to eat dinner no later than 7:30 PM for the next two weeks. Try 7:00 PM for the following two weeks after that.

In addition, get in the habit of brushing your teeth right after dinner. This may help prevent you from further snacking. Be very mindful about snacking late at night. If you can't seem to get rid of this bad habit, look for the underlying cause; it's not hunger for food.

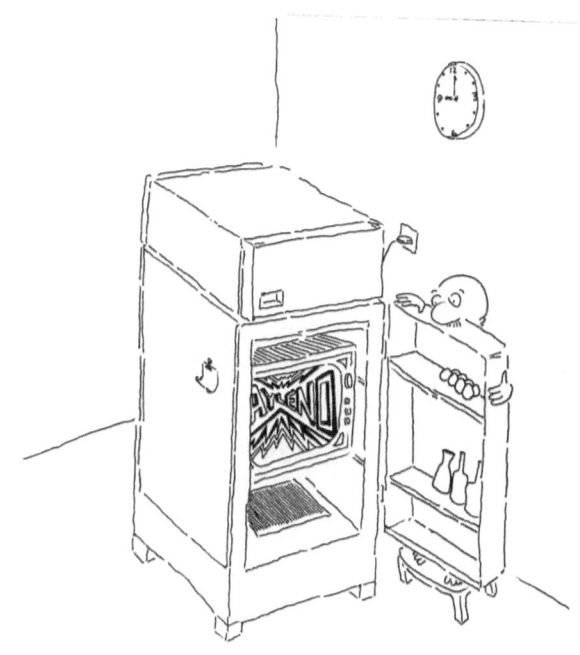

Chapter 10

Minimize ACNFFPD Consumption

You are the sum total of everything
you've ever done to yourself.
—biochemist and cancer researcher Ernst T. Krebs Jr.

What's this, you ask? It means minimize alcohol, caffeine, nicotine, fast food, and pharmaceutical drugs consumption. Duh, that's obvious, you must be saying. Then why are so many people still imbibing? Let's remind ourselves why we need to back off, cut down and, perhaps, stop altogether:

Alcohol: alcohol depletes the body of nutrients. It is a toxin to the body and as such requires liquids to flush out. Alcohol consumption results in dehydration and is a burden to the liver and kidneys, our eliminatory organs.

I highly recommend restricting alcohol consumption to no more than twice weekly. The exception is red wine or beer, which can be consumed about three to four times a week in the amount of one glass of red wine or a small bottle of beer instead.

Caffeine: the most prevalent and popular drug of all. Like alcohol, caffeine is a toxin that depletes your body of nutrients and liquids, leaving you under-nourished and dehydrated. It also increases the load on the kidneys and liver. The worst thing you can do is drink coffee first thing in the morning when your body needs to re-hydrate after seven to eight hours of sleep. If you decide you have to have that cup of coffee anyway, drink a bottle of water too to help your body flush out the toxins and re-hydrate.

As someone who struggles with coffee cravings myself, I recommend restricting consumption of this roller-coaster-inducing drug to no more than once daily. I also recommend you try green tea with honey instead of coffee the next time you walk into Starbucks. Who knows, you might even like it!

Nicotine: smoking is slow suicide. It depletes the body of many nutrients and has been linked to an increased risk of heart disease, lung cancer, and emphysema. When you smoke around a nonsmoker you expose him or her to those same risks, and that is pure selfishness. As someone who smoked a pack a day, from the age of fifteen to the age of thirty, I understand it's not easy to quit. Successfully quitting smoking was one of the hardest things I've ever done and something I'm very proud of. What helped me to quit was a daily yoga practice. Yoga cleanses the blood of toxins, and when your blood is free of nicotine, the craving for this drug drops significantly. So, do yourself a favor; enough with coughing out mucus and smelling and looking like an ashtray. Make a commitment to quit. Don't tell anyone. Don't make declarations. Just put that cigarette box in a drawer and forget about it. Believe me, you will never regret it.

How I quit smoking: when my father, who never smoked, caught me smoking at the age of seventeen, I told him that by the time I was thirty I'd quit smoking. Little did I know then that this prediction would come true or the way it would come to happen. When I was twenty-seven I joined an eight-week yoga for beginners course. At this course I learned a series of movements called "Sun Salutes" designed to be performed in the morning. I started practicing these movements every morning in order to alleviate a herniated disk I was suffering from. But lo and behold, besides relieving the herniated disk, my cravings for cigarettes started diminishing. After a few months I couldn't smoke at all. The yoga exercises helped clean my blood and cells from nicotine, and hence cravings for cigarettes diminished. As a matter of fact, every time I would smoke, besides getting dizzy, I felt a tingling sensation in my feet as if the nicotine circulated through my body. I was nearly thirty years old and indeed it was time to quit. Unlike previous times, this time was for good.

Fast Food: you only have to check out the movies *Super Size Me* and *Fast Food Nation* to understand how detrimental fast food is to your health. Fast food contains high amounts of saturated fats, refined sugars, excess salt, nitrogen, and other chemicals that are hazardous to our health. In many cases hamburgers sold in fast food chains contain fecal matter. I'm not suggesting that you eliminate fast food altogether. If you crave a Big Mac or a Whopper every once in a while, go ahead. Just don't make this kind of toxic food your primary diet. Remember, you are what you eat.

Former FDA commissioner David Kessler talks in his new book *The End of Overeating: Taking Control of the Insatiable American Appetite*, about how tasty foods change your brain, and how the food industry designs the fat, salt, and sugar-laden snacks you crave. Kessler, the former head of the FDA during the Bush and Clinton administrations, claims that part of the blame for the current American overeating plague we are witnessing lies with the food industry. By adding to food the above ingredients they create dependency and cravings. When consuming these altered foods, one is constantly in a vicious cycle of unstable blood sugar levels which creates, as the old Fleetwood Mac song says, *constant cravings*.

Pharmaceutical Drugs: according to the *Centers for Disease control and Prevention* (CDC), recent statistics suggest that drug-related poisoning accidents are second only to motor-vehicle crashes as a cause of unintentional injury deaths in the United States. Fifty people die of unintentional drug overdoses in the United States each day most of which are attributed to psychotherapeutic drugs and prescription narcotic painkillers.[10] And a recent study titled *Death by Medicine* concluded that the number of people having in-hospital, adverse drug reactions (ADR) to prescribed medicine is 2.2 million.[11]

There are a number of reasons for theses staggering statistics. First of all, most pharmaceutical drugs contain toxins. Second, many of them have myriad side effects. Unwittingly combining two non-compatible products (which happens rather frequently) can produce catastrophic results. And finally, continuous consumption of these types of medicines can negatively affect both the liver as well as the lining of both the stomach and the intestines.

You see, the problem with most pharmaceuticals is that they are only intended to treat symptoms, not the root source of the problem. This is sort of like disconnecting the check engine light in your car rather than investigating and repairing the engine problem. I'm not in any way suggesting here that you should avoid pharmaceuticals altogether. Sometimes when you're suffering from acute symptoms,

---

[10] www.cdc.gov/mmwr/preview/mmwrhtml/mm5605a1.htm **February 9, 2007 / 56(05); 93–96.**

[11] *Death by Medicine* by Gary Null, PhD Carolyn Dean, MD, ND Martin Feldman, MD Debora Rasio, MD Dorothy Smith, PhD, 2003.

pharmaceuticals can offer great relief. But they should never be the solution to any ongoing medical or physical discomfort. Treat the root cause of the problem, not the symptoms.

Getting in the Habit

For the next couple of weeks be mindful about consuming any of the above products. Choose one and make a conscious decision to cut its consumption by half. Stick with it for a while and then cut it by half again. Repeat this with the next item and the next.

In a year's time, you should be a less toxic person and feeling great about it.

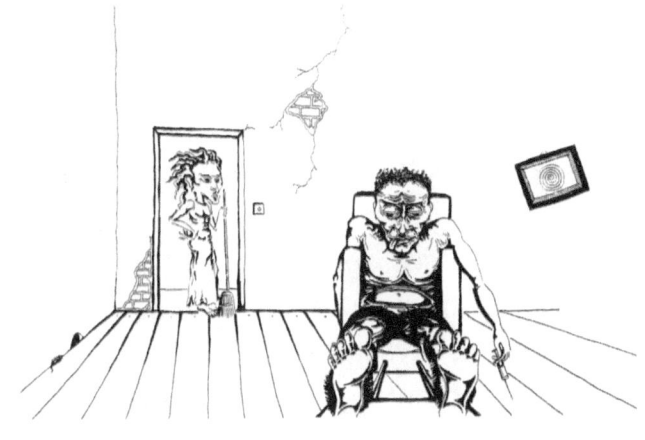

Wife: *Joe, what are you doing?*
Joe: *Shooting heroin.*
Wife: *Why ... ?*
Joe: *The book said no coffee, no booze, and no cigarettes. What's left?*

Chapter 11

Peace Within

We can never obtain peace in the outer world
until we make peace with ourselves.
—Dalai Lama

In today's hectic world we are bombarded with stressors on all fronts. From work to colleagues, clients, and bosses to traffic and siblings, and of course, our immediate relationships, we face a mass of demands and pressures. It can get to the point that you feel like screaming: *stop the world, I want to get off!*

Well, believe or not, you *can* stop the world and get off. All you need is a quiet place to center yourself and calm your mind. And one of the best ways to achieve this state is meditation.

There are many forms of meditation, from transcendental meditation to active meditation and guided imagery.

Studies have shown that meditation helps increase concentration and focus, lower blood pressure, and contribute to an overall feeling of well-being and confidence.

One form of meditation I'm very fond of is the *Silva Life System*. You can learn more about Silva method at www.silvalifesystem.com

Another way to learn meditation is by joining a local yoga center. Most of them teach meditation, and you can learn the basics there and then continue on your own. In addition, most yoga classes start and end with a wonderful relaxation routine that can be very beneficial. The practice of yoga itself is a form of active meditation, which helps quiet the mind and prepare it for passive meditation.

If you don't feel comfortable with any of these suggestions, there are other forms of meditation and relaxation you can adopt. Hiking or just spending time in nature can have a deep, relaxing, and soothing effect on the mind, body, and soul. Gardening, cooking, listening to music, playing an instrument, or adopting any kind of hobby are all forms of relaxation and meditation.

According to a January 2, 2009, article in the *Boston Globe* titled *How the City Hurts Your Brain,* by Jonah Lehrer, recent studies suggest that although the *city* has always been an engine of intellectual life, from the eighteenth-century coffeehouses of London, where citizens gathered to discuss chemistry and radical politics, to the Left Bank bars of modern Paris, where Pablo Picasso held forth on modern art, constant exposure to urban life and lack of exposure to nature can impair brain function. According to scientists, just being in an urban environment impairs our basic mental processes. After spending a few minutes on a crowded city street, the brain is less able to hold things in memory and suffers from reduced self-control. This new research suggests that cities actually dull our thinking, sometimes dramatically so. In contrast, just having a glimpse of nature can dramatically improve brain function. Studies have demonstrated, for instance, that hospital patients recover more quickly when they can see trees from their windows and that women living in public housing are better able to focus when their apartment overlooks a grassy courtyard. Natural settings are full of objects that automatically capture our attention, yet without triggering a negative emotional response—unlike, say, a backfiring car. The mental machinery that directs attention can relax deeply and replenish itself when absorbed in nature.

Sleep, the Ultimate Relaxation

Another important form of relaxation is getting a good night's sleep. According to a 2005 Sleep in America Poll, 75 percent of Americans report that they have trouble sleeping on a regular basis. It's very hard to be effective during the day if you can't rest and rejuvenate at night.

Here are a few tips to help you get a good night's sleep:

- According to Ayurveda, the five-thousand-year-old Indian science of life, health, and longevity, everything in nature is cyclical, including each day. According to Ayurveda, the best time to go to sleep is two to three hours after sundown. This translates to between 8:00 and 11:00 PM, depending on the season. For most of us 8:00 PM or even 9:00 PM is way too early to go to bed. But if you consistently having difficulty falling asleep, I highly recommend that you try going to bed around 10:00 to 11:00 PM on regular basis, and no later than 12:00 AM.

- Avoid caffeinated drinks after 4:00 or 5:00 PM and restrict caffeine consumption to no more than one drink per day.

- Meditate before going to sleep; this will help you calm your nerves and mind and allow you to release the day's stressful events and thoughts.

- Weather permitting, take an evening stroll. It's another great way to leave the day's events behind.

- Take a warm bath or shower before going to bed, preferably with aroma-therapeutic lavender scent.

- Read a relaxing book

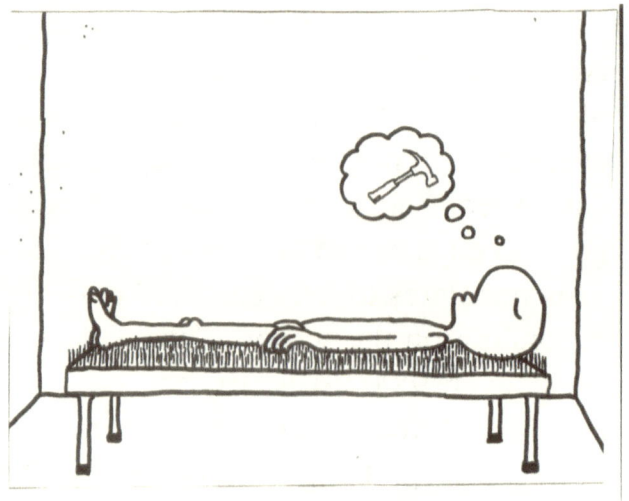

Sweet Dreams

As you start to use the method(s) of relaxation and rejuvenation that suits you best, you'll gradually start to notice that your body and mind are working in sync, and your life flows more easily. You'll be able to "stop the world" at will, and get back on with less stress to enjoy the rest of life's magnificent ride.

Getting in the Habit

Choose one of the relaxation methods recommended above. Put it into practice for the next week. If you decide to adopt a meditation practice, find a yoga center in your area and join their classes. Make a commitment to practice your relaxation method at least fifteen minutes every day. When the week is over, make a commitment to continue for one more week. It usually takes twenty-one days to adopt a new habit, so keep going for one more week.

Chapter 12

Soul Food—Our Primary Nourishment

Twenty years from now you will be more disappointed by the things you didn't do than by the ones you did do. So throw off the bowlines. Sail away from the safe harbor. Catch the trade winds in your sails. Explore. Dream. Discover.
—Mark Twain

The physical food we eat is fuel for our vehicle (body). But as with any road trip, the driver (our soul) requires nourishment as well. The food our soul craves is love, fulfillment, joy, and spirituality. So, if you're unfulfilled at your job, get another one. If you don't have somebody to love, find someone. Make the time to simply have fun. And celebrate every day as if it were your last. Life is truly too short, so enjoy it to the last drop.

Meditating on Solutions

On a more serious note, many eating disorders and even illnesses can result from dissatisfaction in certain areas of our lives. It could be dissatisfaction with work, marriage life, immediate relationships, or simply boredom. Whatever it might be, if there is a problem, I highly recommend trying to identify the source of your discontent and then finding ways to resolve it. It may not be easy, but neglecting life problems can have disastrous effects on your health. I personally believe that identifying the root cause of a problem is half the solution, and facing it head on is far better than sweeping it under the rug.

Joshua Rosenthal, head of The Institute for Integrative Nutrition in New York City, describes how he stumbled upon the concept of primary food: "The importance of primary food became abundantly clear to me when I started a natural food store in Toronto. Sometimes after I closed the store at night, I would go to the movie theatre next door, where I noticed that many of the popcorn-munching, soda-gulping moviegoers looked happier and healthier than many of my customers. It became obvious to me that food was only half of the equation when it came to creating health. Eating well helps, but don't expect it to work miracles. It can fill you, but it cannot fulfill you."

In my own experience one of the best ways I've found to identify the solution to any challenge in my life is by utilizing a meditation practice. Meditation helps you to see things clearly and can guide you to solutions by calming and focusing your mind.

Vitamin L

I also believe hobbies are crucial to our soul's well-being. Doing something you like or love helps you to forget about the rest of the world for a while and time flies. A hobby also offers a sense of fulfillment and can rejuvenate your life. Those lucky few who manage to turn their hobby into a career are truly blessed; after all, they never have to get up for "work."

Home cooking is another important aspect of soul food. When you cook at home, you not only gain control over the ingredients that go into the food, but you also add one very key ingredient—*love*, or as I like to call it, vitamin L. Vitamin L is one vitamin we can never have enough of.

Getting in the Habit

For the next week make a decision to eat in at least once a day. In addition, take time to perform an inventory check and identify the areas in your life you are not satisfied with. Once you identify an area, make a list of possible solutions. You may need a few hours or even days to complete this exercise, but stick with it. Once you have all of your possible solutions listed, pick the one that resonates with you the most. Put it into practice at once! Once you get the ball rolling, strange and wonderful things will happen. It may not always be what you intended, but I can assure you the risk will be worth taking.

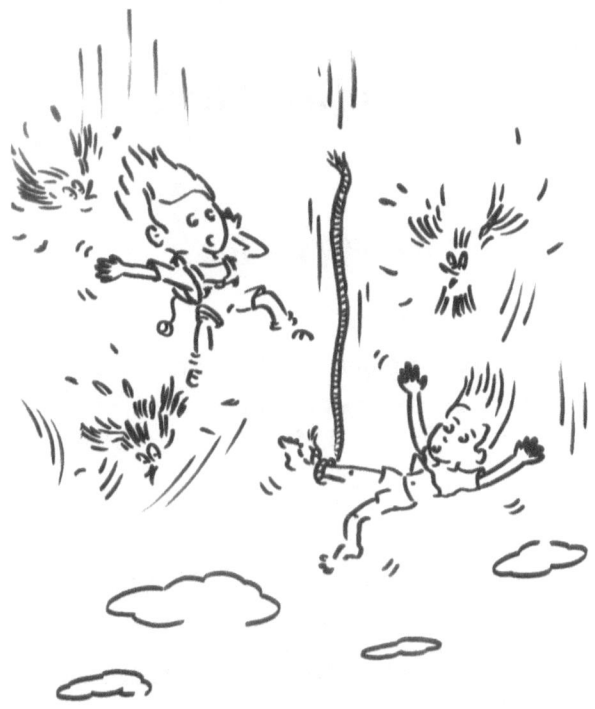

A. *Isn't bungee jumping fun?*

B. *This is skydiving, not bungee jumping, and where is your parachute anyway?*

A. *Oh, don't worry, this is a strong cord, I'm sure I'll bounce back ...*

Chapter 13

The 90/10 Rule

*Our greatest glory is not in never falling
but in rising every time we fall.*
—Confucius

Let's face it, no one's perfect. Not even the Dalai Lama. The 90/10 rule states that what you do most of the time (or 90 percent) has a bigger impact on your life than what you do every once in a while (or 10 percent). We can try to be good 90 percent of the time and let go the other 10 percent.

For example, let's say that you're out for dinner at a fancy restaurant, and your mouth is salivating over the filet mignon in red wine reduction served with lobster mashed potato. What a treat! But wait! *You can't mix meat with potatoes, proteins with carbs!* Forget about it! That's right, have fun and enjoy yourself. Tomorrow you'll get back on the wagon and make sure you eat properly for the rest of the week. It's okay to "sin" once in a while, 10 percent of the time, in fact, as long as we adhere to a proper diet and healthy lifestyle the other 90 percent of the time. Our bodies have an extraordinary capability of healing themselves when nourished on a daily basis.

I know the 90/10 principle seems to contradict the rest of this book. But there's a concrete reason for this "release valve." If you are anything like me, chances are as soon as you finish reading this book you'll immediately try to adopt each of the preceding principles—to the letter. Since you are a human, there's an equally good chance that you won't be able to maintain the changes for a prolonged period of time and will start slacking off. This can lead to feeling guilty and thoughts like: "Oh, I mixed proteins and carbs today," or "Oh no, I ate after 8:00 PM," which, in turn, leads to stress and resentment.

Since people don't like to feel this way, they'll often opt for the easiest solution; quitting their new lifestyle altogether and going back to their unhealthy habits.

The purpose of the 90/10 rule is to prevent this entire self-defeating scenario from happening in the first place. What's important is what you do *most* of the time. And it's really all about maintaining a healthy *balance* between healthy living and letting go. The more informed you are the better choices you can make, which means when you do slack off, at least you are aware enough to know what commitments you have to make to your own *body* in order to balance the effects.

> According to T. Harv Ecker, author of the number one *NY Times* best-seller *Secrets of the Millionaire Mind,* one reason that people don't achieve what they want in life is that they make commitments they don't keep or they don't commit at all. For example, say you made a New Year's resolution to lose weight and as a result made a commitment to work out in the gym four times a week. The only trouble is that you currently work out zero to one times a week. You may be able to keep this commitment for a week or two, but it will be hard for most people to sustain this level if they didn't do it before. As soon as we lapse on our commitments, deep inside we feel failure; we said we would do something and we didn't. By all means this is a failure, and no one likes to feel this way. So when this happens frequently enough, we cease to make meaningful commitments and the result of that is that we don't get anywhere. The secret, according to Mr. Ecker, is to make commitments that will challenge you and at the same time, you know are achievable. If we go back to the same example, say you commit to attend the gym two to three times a week for the next two weeks. This is challenging (you only went zero to one times per week prior), yet is achievable.

At the end of these two weeks, assuming you kept this commitment, you may challenge yourself again; this time commit to attend three to four times a week for the following two weeks. And once you accomplish this commitment, commit to attend at least four times per week the next two weeks.

This process of making commitments and keeping them will make you feel more confident and successful. And everybody likes to feel successful. By setting short-term goals and achieving them you create a positive and pleasurable experience for yourself, rather than that of feeling guilt, self-resentment, and defeat, an experience that will make you move forward.

Getting in the Habit

One of the best ways to make sure the 90/10 rule doesn't become the 50/50 rule is by tracking everything you eat. By that I don't mean necessarily counting calories (I don't believe our ancestors were walking around counting calories all day long), but rather being aware of what you put on your plate. For example, if you are away on a business trip and forced to eat in a restaurant that doesn't serve the healthiest food, you can always choose fish instead of hamburger, chicken instead of steak, and salad instead of fries or mashed potato. If your dish comes with cheese, ask for it without. If you are used to having breakfast at Starbucks, ask for oatmeal or a bran muffin instead of refined scones; at least you'll get some fiber in your diet. These little changes can make all the difference between a healthy and not-so-healthy meal.

The bottom line is as long as you maintain a healthy lifestyle 90 percent of the time, it's okay to loosen up and have fun the other 10 percent. You'll probably even appreciate it more.

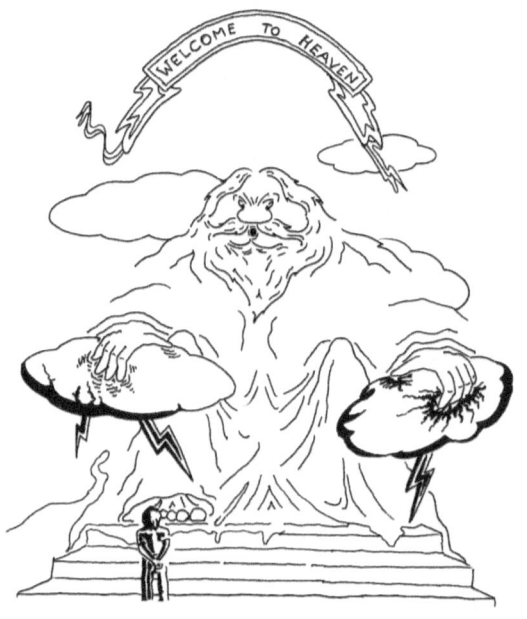

God: *Why should I let you in to heaven?*

Joe: *I was good 90 percent of the time.*

God: *And what did you do the other 10 percent?*

Joe: *Party like there's no tomorrow!*

Last Things Last

Time and health are two precious assets that we don't
recognize and appreciate until they have been depleted.
—Denis Waitley, Self-Mastery Expert

As we come to the end of this book I'd like to share a few final words. This book was intended to be a light and easy introduction to the world of balanced nutrition and healthy lifestyles. As such it cannot provide in-depth information on these topics. If you'd like to dive deeper into the world of holistic health and nutrition, I suggest you take a look at the resources page and select a couple of books from that list.

Remember, unlike your car, you only have one body to take you through life. The more attentive you are to your body and the earlier you start maintaining it properly, the better your "ride" will be in later years. And isn't this what life is all about? Experiencing a great, adventurous, satisfying, and pleasurable ride?

So, be mindful, make good choices when it comes to the food you eat, treat your body well, and by God, *enjoy your life!*

I leave you with one last quote from Dr. Wayne Dyer, "Habits are changed by practicing new behavior, and this is true for mental habits as well."

Resources

Rogers A. R., Lltis D., and Wooding S., 2004. Genetic variation at the MC1R locus and the time since loss of human body hair. *Current Anthropology*, 45(1): 105–108.

D'Adamo, Dr. Peter J. *Eat Right for Your Type*. Tel Aviv: Hoop-A-J00p, LLC, 1997.

Day, Phillip. *Health Wars*. Kent, England: Credence Publications, 2001.

Douillard, John. *The 3-Season Diet*. New York: Three Rivers Press, 2000.

Fleckenstein, MD, Alexa and Weisman, Roanne. *Own Your Health, Healthy to 100*. Deerfield Beach, Florida: Health Communications, Inc. 2006.

Global College of Natural Medicine Study Guide. Santa Cruz, California: GCNM, 2004–2005.

Godagama, Dr. Shantha. *The Handbook of Ayurveda*. Boston, Massachusetts: Journy Editions, 1998.

Holford, Patrick. *The New Optimum Nutrition Bible*. London: Piatkus Books, 1997.

Kessler, MD, David. *The End of Overeating: Taking Control of the Insatiable American Appetite*. New York: Rodale Books, 2009.

Khan, MSc, Sara Anees, et. al. *Nutrition, the International Journal of Applied and Basic Nutritional Sciences*, Volume 23, Issue 9, September 2007.

Lad, Dr. Vasant. *Ayurveda, the Science of Self-Healing.* Twin Lakes, Wisconsin: Lotus Press, 1990.

Francis M. Pottenger, Jr. *Pottenger's Cats: A Study in Nutrition.* Lemon Grove, CA Price-Pottenger Nutrition Foundation Inc. *1995.*

Reid, Daniel P. *The Tao of Health, Sex and Longevity.* New York: Simon & Schuster, 1989

Rosenthal, Joshua. *Integrative Nutrition Study Guide.* New York: Integrative Nutrition Publishing, 2006.

Weil, MD, Andrew. *Eight Weeks to Optimum Health.* New York: Alfred A. Knopf, 1997.